Confronting Theory

In olden days a glimpse of theory
Was looked on as something dreary
Now, Heaven knows,
Anything goes!

Apologies to Cole Porter

Does it contain any experimental reasoning
concerning fact and existence?
No. Well, don't commit it to the flames, all the same;
but *be careful.*

David Hume

Confronting Theory
The Psychology of Cultural Studies

Philip Bell

intellect Bristol, UK / Chicago, USA

First published in the UK in 2010 by
Intellect, The Mill, Parnall Road, Fishponds, Bristol, BS16 3JG, UK

First published in the USA in 2010 by
Intellect, The University of Chicago Press, 1427 E. 60th Street,
Chicago, IL 60637, USA

Copyright © 2010 Intellect Ltd

All rights reserved. No part of this publication may be reproduced,
stored in a retrieval system, or transmitted, in any form or by
any means, electronic, mechanical, photocopying, recording, or
otherwise, without written permission.

A catalogue record for this book is available from the
British Library.

Cover designer: Holly Rose
Copy-editor: Heather Owen
Typesetting: Mac Style, Beverley, E. Yorkshire

ISBN 978-1-84150-317-2

Contents

Preface	7
Chapter 1: Cultural Studies and Capital-T Theory	13
Chapter 2: What is Theory About?	29
Chapter 3: Different Things	41
Chapter 4: Theory, People and 'Subjects'	57
Chapter 5: 'Post-Human' Theory and Cultural Studies	71
Chapter 6: Affecting Ontologies	87
Chapter 7: Real experience, Un-real Science	105
Chapter 8: Theory and Education	123
References	141
Index	145

Preface

> There is not a fixed and yet there is a common, human nature: without the latter there would be no possibility of talking about human beings, or, indeed, of communication, on which all thought depends – and not only thought, but feeling, imagination, action. (Berlin [1986] 2004: 26)

In the twenty-plus years since Isaiah Berlin wrote this 'letter on human nature', a lot has changed, including what it means to write a letter. More significantly, of course, the idea that humans 'have' a nature, and that academic disciplines need to understand this if they are to converse about communication, imagination and feelings, sounds quaintly 'essentialist' and indefensibly 'humanist' in today's post-disciplinary academy.

The eight essays in this book address overlapping aspects of the theoretical assumption that human experience, culture, communication, and 'life' itself can be meaningfully understood without reference to 'human nature' (however flexible and non-essentialist that concept may be). I present arguments against the idea that systematic empirical knowledge about people, their biology and their psychology, is irrelevant to the domains of the humanities [sic] and social sciences. I regard it as educationally imperative that students be taught that it is possible to know objective things about why and how people behave and feel as they do in particular cultural and social circumstances. I mount this thesis by examining key concepts and assumptions in post-humanist capital-T Theory: is it epistemologically and ontologically more tenable, more productive, more useful as the basis for conversing about cultural life than the episteme that it overturns?

Darwin, Marx, Freud, even in their own different ways, Piaget, Skinner, Levi-Strauss and Judith Butler – all describe dimensions of social and psychological life and assumed that human beings were an animal species with certain qualities, capacities, dispositions and physical limitations. Amongst other things they disagreed about what kinds of explanatory (and that meant *causal*) accounts of different human lives needed to be postulated to understand various human interactions, their biology, social histories, and multiple, ever-changing cultures. But all these writers assumed that the different phenomena and processes they were trying to understand were real: they made competing, but contestable claims about what is the case. They adopted publicly defined terminologies, however novel they may have been at the time (e.g. Freud's 'cathexes', Marx's 'surplus value') and were not immune to theoretical analysis – they were certainly not naïvely anti-theory, not naïve 'positivists' (Skinner, perhaps, excluded). For my purposes, however, the most important methodological assumption that united all those who theorized about people and studied them empirically within the social and biological sciences, was that they each understood that they could have been in error, and if so, they *could be shown to be in error*.

From the 1970s at least, European philosophical writings increasingly competed with empirico-realist epistemologies in Anglo-American humanities and social science curricula. Few methodological certainties remained by the end of the century as students learned to question realism, reductionism, essentialism, and Western epistemological 'foundationalism'. New '-isms' and '-ologies' peppered academic discourse, questioning the assumed objectivity of knowledge ('scientific' knowledge included). In fact, as will be discussed in this book, humanities students today are very likely to leave university equipped with an armoury of arguments against science's claim to objectivity, whether or not they have attained even rudimentary knowledge of any particular science during their own studies. (Ironically, graduates from science faculties are unlikely to know anything at all about these 'critical paradigms').

I believe that post-disciplinary education in what is now called 'Cultural Studies' has not earned the right to such dismissive anti-realist complacency. Theory-inspired Cultural Studies has shown too little regard for cogency, coherence, truth and evidence. In mounting its attacks on the very possibility of knowing things about people, Cultural Studies writers have often ignored the liberating demands of reason and objectivity. As a result they have denied students the opportunity to converse with each other about common cultural, political and social issues. If all knowledge is completely language-dependent (or 'theory-dependent') in the strong sense of these terms – if novel realities can be invoked through words alone – knowledge is quickly reduced to mere belief and high-sounding opinion. Epistemological modesty in the face of recalcitrant reality and contingency is not encouraged in such an educational environment.

I find it ironic to have written this book. I am at best a 'lapsed psychologist', having taught in the media and cultural fields for almost four decades, the period of the ascent of post-disciplinary studies. And I have a long history of critically analysing essentialism and reductionism (for instance, in regard to representations of gender and 'race'). I have been consistently critical of the methodological and educational triviality of much of academic psychology itself.[1] I have maintained a consistently anti-reductionist and anti-positivist position. In fact, forty years ago I wrote an undergraduate essay that argued against the logical possibility of reducing psychological predicates to physiological descriptors. Mental phenomena could not be understood nor explained only as physico-chemical phenomena, but had to be defined relationally. Any coherent account of consciousness had to allow that consciousness was always 'of' some state of affairs that existed independently of the brain.

Fast forward to the new millennium – today I have been forced to restate these kinds of arguments in the context of the saturation of what is now called Cultural Studies 'discourse' by ad hoc psychological concepts and metaphysical postulates so abstract that only dogs can hear them, as students often joke. As a university teacher, I have tried to comfort my bemused and confused charges with counter arguments to the new-fangled idealisms and metaphysical houses of cards that 'Theory'-writers have constructed.

As I no longer have teaching responsibilities, nor carry the soul-destroying burden of administering a large academic unit, I have taken the opportunity to confront several aspects of 'Theory', asking that its proponents justify their methodological assumptions and metaphysical excesses. I try to break out of the circular corral of textuality and the question-begging defence of inter-textuality. Instead, I ask what the claims of particular cultural Theory analyses of psychological issues imply – what could each mean, if anything, empirically. I briefly outline the relevance of the analyses I canvass to psychological issues (for example, to questions of human emotions, when I deal with 'affect'), and sketch some of the relevant historical contexts from which Theory and Anglo-American academic psychology both developed.

I have tried to be fair to examples of writing that I admit I sometimes find pretentious and affected, by taking their authors 'at their word', so to speak. I have laboured over many texts that yielded very little enlightenment, but have done so in good faith, hoping to understand them before offering my critique. In this I have acknowledged the respective writers' own advice that their analyses are not meant to be interpreted figuratively (e.g. metaphorically), but are intended to be read literally. I have tried not to be dismissive, even though I judge many analyses found in Cultural Studies to be philosophically naïve. This has meant that I have included many lengthy quotations from works popular with Cultural Studies academics and hence likely to be familiar to students. Although I have limited my technically philosophical arguments, the educational issues that agitate my concern do demand some epistemological sophistication of my readers at times. So where appropriate I have explained what is at stake in technical terms, I hope clearly enough for undergraduate readers and their teachers alike to understand. And I have resisted the temptation to satirize the examples I discuss (well, mostly), although I have done so elsewhere in less formal contexts, I have to confess.[2]

It will be clear from the above that this is not a book about culture or cultures. It is concerned with the psychological and philosophical assumptions woven into what is referred to today as 'Theory'. Theory both subtends and ornaments the otherwise prosaic, descriptive and critical writing that in Anglo-American post-disciplinary education is usually labelled 'Cultural Studies'.

Although the term 'postmodernism' is freely and pejoratively circulated in today's academy, I have tried to avoid it. 'Postmodernity' as a socio-cultural period, or as a label for computer-age aesthetics ('after' modernism), is misleadingly vague when applied to educational/philosophical paradigms, even though the examples I deal with have also flourished during the past quarter of a century. I am interested in Cultural Studies' complacent disregard of any technically precise methodology from the fields it cannibalizes and rewrites.

The eight overlapping essays are my attempt to encourage methodological modesty and to reinstate realist coherence as a 'default' position in the post-disciplinary humanities and social sciences, at least in regard to what most people would accept to be psychological matters. By 'psychological' I mean pertaining to the mental, emotional and behavioural lives of (human) beings, although I am aware that other species may offer comparative insights about human psychology, and even about culture. In fact, one Cultural Studies luminary discusses perception in relation to honeybees, so I consider this unexpected example in one chapter.

Confronting Theory may be read as a series of independent analyses of constellations of related concepts nowadays fashionable within Cultural Studies. Or it can be used as a set of critical arguments in which the educational implications of Theory-speak and the plea for a reinvigorated humanist realism in the humanities and social sciences are the linking themes. So I have countenanced some repetitions to allow Chapters 2 to 7 each to be read separately. My concerns are educational, and therefore necessarily methodological or philosophical.

Thanks are due to many students (especially my chronically-confused Honours level students from seminars dealing with methodological issues in Media/Cultural Studies), and to those colleagues prepared to debate the assumptions ingrained in their own work (which is not a lot, unsurprisingly). Dr Mark Milic and Dr Fiona Hibberd have been especially encouraging and insightful. Fiona Hibberd's rigorous and comprehensive *Unfolding Social Constructionism* (2005) has become an invaluable resource for me during the preparation of my book. It forensically dissects perennial debates about language, psychology and epistemology, arguing for the necessity of realism against language-dependent relativisms. These are issues I necessarily canvass as part of my analyses of Theory's ambitious metaphysics, but I have other, more recent debates to address, and I do not pretend to emulate Hibberd's philosophical sophistication.

My research has been supported by the Faculty of Arts and Social Sciences, at the University of New South Wales, Sydney. Marie McKenzie's diligence and professionalism as my research assistant have been invaluable, and Dr John Golder has subjected my every sentence to sophisticated editorial scrutiny (I now think I know when to use dashes rather than parentheses, as a result). Of course, any errors of fact or limitations of argument are mine, and I look forward to discussion of the issues I raise by those consoled, provoked or offended by what I hope is a rigorous series of analyses. Above all, I hope that students who have found themselves marooned on the island of Cultural Studies will use this book to build a dwelling sturdy enough to withstand the tidal waves of idealist fashion. They might even discover that the tsunami that intimidates them is no more than a sea mirage after all.

Note: neologisms, spelling and capitalization

Readers of *Confronting Theory* may be confounded by many of the novel terms that currently circulate in Cultural Studies. Wherever possible I have implicitly (or explicitly) defined these. I hope that I have conveyed the import of the various neologisms and novel uses of conventional English words by locating them as carefully as space allows in their post-disciplinary contexts.

Where I refer to an established academic discipline, like Psychology or Biology, I have capitalized its name. And, of course, I follow the post-disciplinary convention of calling the kind of writing I discuss as capital-T Theory ('Theory' for short).

Australian spelling follows (generally) British conventions rather than North American. However, I have not altered quotes, nor felt it necessary to note this in every case. I have tried to resist the temptation to exclaim '*sic*' (thus, or 'as in the original' text that I am considering, however startling an excerpt or neologism) but I have had to include occasional warnings to remind readers that I have not fabricated the texts I criticize.

Notes

1. Psychology is good: true/false, *Australian Psychologist*, 1978, 13(2), 211–218; P Bell and P Staines *Logical Psych: Reasoning, Explanation and writing in Psychology*, 2001, Sydney, UNSW Press, 2001. Published in UK and USA by Sage Publications, UK, as *Evaluating, Doing and Writing Research in Psychology*, 2001, (with J Michell).
2. For example, *What's Left of Theory? Deleuzians of Grandeur* (available from p.bell@unsw.edu.au).

Chapter 1

Cultural Studies and Capital-T Theory

The desire to understand the world is, they think, an outdated folly.
Bertrand Russell

The Problem of 'Theory'

Five hundred years have elapsed since Erasmus complained that the writings of his contemporaries were '[f]ull of big words, and newly invented terms ... [a] wall of imposing definitions, conclusions, corollaries, and explicit and implicit propositions protects them' (Erasmus [1509]2008). Clearly, a Renaissance scholar could not have anticipated the rise of the empirical sciences, including social sciences such as Psychology. On the other hand, Erasmus might not have been surprised to learn that obscure rhetoric and opaque neologisms confound students in the twenty-first century as readily as they did in the sixteenth.

Of the various strands of meta-theory in Anglophone interdisciplinary writing that melds the humanities and the social sciences, anti-realist epistemology, arbitrary relativisms and, most recently, the assumption of 'new realities' have re-emerged as the most dominant. Today, students of Cultural Studies are asked to read and write about 'infra-empirical' phenomena, about processes of such abstraction that they seem to refer to no material entities, such as 'affect', 'becomings' and 'intensities'. Sometimes these terms are referred to as 'concepts', although they often lack precise definition. They sound like many terms found in the vocabulary of academic psychology, but they are seldom used in psychologically realist ways – or so I propose to argue in the pages that follow.

I want to begin with a paragraph of prose by a prominent Cultural Studies Theorist. I am aware that I am presenting it out of context, and I shall return later to consider its source in detail. For the moment it is meant only to illustrate the linguistic ecstasy that is common in 'Theory' writing – writing that *purports* to be about real psychological processes, situations and events, and therefore to *refer to* actual phenomena. The author appears to be discussing emotion and 'affect'. And it is not unfair, I think, to say that he *invokes* psychological-sounding terms to create a kind of incantatory effect. His field is perennial issues in academic psychology: here he defines what, following the philosophers Spinoza and Deleuze, he calls 'affect'. Now, please read on, but slowly:

> Reserve the term 'emotion' for the personalized content, and affect for its continuation. Emotion is contextual. Affect is situational: event fully ingressive into context. Serially so: affect is trans-situational. As processional it is precessional, affect inhabits the passage ... It [affect] is pre- and post-contextual, pre- and post-personal, an excess of continuity invested only in the ongoing: its own. Self-continuity across the gaps. Impersonal affect is

the continuing thread of experience. It is the invisible glue that holds the world together. In event. The world-glue of affect is an autonomy of event-connection continuing across its own serialized capture in context. (Massumi 2002: 217)

I shall return to this kind of psychological-sounding capital-T Theory in later chapters. Let me merely note here that this passage is typical of the book from which it is taken, a monograph hailed by many prominent Cultural Studies academics as a 'brilliant achievement', 'an extraordinary work of scholarship'. Significantly, for my concerns in what follows, another prominent cultural Theorist, Isabel Stengers, praises Brian Massumi's work as continuing the 'great radical-empiricist protest against naïve objectivism and naïve subjectivism ... bringing wonder back into everyday experience.'

Immediately after the passage quoted above, Massumi explores the metaphysical problem of the subject/object distinction. I want to quote this passage too, as it illustrates the way in which Theory writing often presents philosophical positions (here, on epistemological and ontological issues) as part of its casually-personified, reader-friendly profundity:

The true duality is not the metaphysical opposition between the subject and object. Subject and object always come together in context. They tightly embrace each other in their reciprocal definition in discourse, as the owner and the ownable of conventional content. The true duality is between continuity and discontinuity (trans-situation and context). This is not a metaphysical opposition. It is processural rhythm, in and of the world, expressing an ontological tension between manipulable objectivity and elusive ongoing qualitative activity (becoming). (Massumi 2002: 217)

Although a work of Cultural Studies and 'Theory' – I shall return to these labels – this book addresses epistemological issues (of objectivism, empiricism, etc.) and postulates a novel kind of ontological realm (which consists of processes rather than objects, for example). Such an ontology seems to demand of the hapless undergraduate sophisticated knowledge of both analytical (Anglo-American) philosophy and European traditions, especially of Bergson and those French writers of the 1960s and 1970s labelled 'post-structuralist'. But, unsurprisingly, few, if any, *post*graduates, let alone undergraduates in cross-disciplinary studies, can claim such erudition. It is more than likely that students reading Massumi in *Cultural Studies 301* would quote without understanding and engage in a kind of academic 'bluffing' that commits them to uncritical acceptance of Theory's metaphysics. Alternatively, they may just turn away, adopting instead the naïve epistemologies that Massumi and his commentators deride.

It is not just students who are befuddled and intimidated by such Theory, by the background knowledge it assumes – and, of course, in Massumi's case, by the willful failure to specify grammatical subjects for the predicates he invents. The cross-disciplinary academic teacher is also likely to feel weak at the knees when reading such intimidating verbiage. But they can at least seek help at conferences that deal with the epistemological paradigm shift that seems to have revolutionized the humanities during the past two decades: 'While the myth of knowledge as objective appears to have been debunked, a question remains unresolved: if not objective, then what?' This teasing question publicized a 2006 conference entitled 'Inside Knowledge'. The blurb went on to discuss the epistemological options facing current transdisciplinary scholarship:

> [A]cademic disciplines today often find themselves trapped between relativist and essentialist tendencies. Faced with the new multiple and complex realities of globalization, cross-cultural encounters and conflicts, the inadequacy of old approaches to knowledge underscores the need for radical revisions of traditional modes of knowledge production, or alternative ways of doing and thinking knowledge. Disciplines therefore appear to be in need of specific methodologies, which could function across disciplinary borders and provide (tentative) grounds for inter- or trans-disciplinary communication. ('Inside Knowledge' Conference 2006)

New ways of 'doing and thinking knowledge' sound pretty exciting: the invitation to throw out the old disciplines of the twentieth-century academy is hard to resist. Yet this challenge to academics working across the humanities assumes no more than what has become conventional wisdom in English-language Arts faculties in the new millennium: *pace* Massumi, this wisdom includes the following:

- All knowledge claims are relative to those making them
- Epistemological certainty based on empirical observation and generalization is a charade
- Only theoretical or conceptually-grounded *interpretation* is possible

This is because

- The foundations of Western metaphysics, including the assumed reality of the psychological subject, are untenable.

The day-to-day context in which students study culture, the media, sociological theory, and in which they must make psychological assumptions about the people who embody culture, has become a theoretical minefield. Even teachers can make only guarded, self-conscious propositions about what is the case. Many fear that their naïvely 'realist' versions of what it means for a person to 'know' something are philosophically untenable. Nor are they wrong to be intimidated about their metaphysical correctness. Analysts like Massumi write as though actual people who think they know something about pre-existing material phenomena, people who believe that the world is populated by more or less permanent material entities, are philosophically ignorant. Like realist social scientists, they are fundamentally mistaken about what exists (their tacit *ontology*) and naïve about how to justify their claims to know or describe it (their *epistemology*). Old-fashioned disciplines may even be judged as *unethical* because they necessarily 'objectify' (or, as Theory has it, 'essentialize') people and other phenomena. By contrast, Theory provides the conceptual apparatus for criticizing and re-writing the humanities and social sciences that became established in Anglophone universities from the 1950s.

So, the 'Inside Knowledge' conference blurb challenges new millennium academics to 'perform' or 'do' knowledge (or 'knowledge' in quotation marks) differently. They must practise 'capital-T Theory'. As I shall demonstrate throughout this book, this practice may take many forms, but most involve developing conceptual abstractions that do not refer directly to any actual things or situations in the world. Rather they designate at best other concepts by which to interpret other interpretations (as 'texts'). This limited aspiration follows not only from the idea that 'unmediated' knowledge of the material world is impossible, but also from the assumption that knowledge claims, being verbal, are usually, if not always, exclusively about language itself. So 'extreme' – or, as I call it, 'ecstatic' – Theory refers to those modes of writing that propose conceptualizations whose metaphysical orientations must be accepted on faith by undergraduates.

Theory offers largely self-referring bodies of abstract concepts and propositions. Rather than low-level *theories* in the plural, such as, say, Freudian theory or Marxist historical accounts of the factors causing the rise of fascism, capital-T Theory presents radically different ways of writing. Theory returns to what, in other technical vocabularies, are more or less empirical terms, but its proponents make few original proposals about what is the case. This is because 'what is the case' is assumed as a kind of 'given', albeit a given that social scientists and traditional scholars misunderstand. To enlighten them, Theory asks that its texts be read as revelations of unexpected dimensions of 'the real' (usually in scare quotes so as not to imply naïvety), or of new relations amongst Theory's own terms. Without recourse to observation of anything other than 'texts', by means of analysis and creative invention of concepts, Theorists mount new arguments about what their readers think they already know, what they take for granted or accept as 'commonsense'.

Sometimes, for example when the narratives known as the 'Oedipus complex' are rewritten as a kind of general theory of human 'un-freedom', as accounts of universal 'oppression' by language or by ideology themselves, one can see a kind of general empirical claim being made. But Theory in Cultural Studies contexts usually 'rewrites' taken-for-granted concepts and knowledge claims, albeit without any expectation that the new version of the phenomena in question should be tested empirically as an alternative putative 'explanation'. Discussing people's pleasure in music, dance, or the perception and experience of cinematic close-ups can produce a neo-phenomenological exuberance centred on words like 'intensity', 'affect' or 'faciality'. These are posed as illuminating concepts, but, as we shall discover in later chapters, their psychological (even their grammatical) status may be unclear at best.

I contend that no method is available to compare the adequacy of one account ("Theory text') against another. This is because Theory (to personify this body of work) refers to modes of writing that ask to be evaluated otherwise than in terms of truth or probability.

This results from the scope of the conceptual assumptions of Theory: its ambition within Cultural Studies seems to be to rewrite the *whole of post-Enlightenment Western metaphysics*. While many have criticized the *epistemological* implications of much that is labelled 'Theory', it is the *ontological assumptions* it imports into Cultural Studies and into the empirical disciplines subsumed by Cultural Studies that render Theory so problematic.

My critique of Theory and of its infiltration into many areas of post-disciplinary discourse will not merely argue that it is sometimes obscure, pretentiously abstract, or conceptually muddled. This may be true – but it would only be a criticism if Theory failed to generate any genuine insights or knowledge. And this is my position: I shall argue that Theory writing becomes hypocritical when its metaphysical 'discourse' sits side by side with more banal claims that rely on the reader assuming the very things that Theory denies, including the physical and psychological reality of actual human beings. I shall try to show that Theory is often no more than an elaborate gloss, or 'translation' into new terms, of the many specific beliefs warranted by evidence and example that are documented in the literature of its disciplinary predecessors in the humanities. These are, of course, the very disciplines that Theory seeks to help students to critique, indeed, to transcend.

'Ecstatic' is the word I use to describe much of the transcendental abstraction that confounds my students. Here is a passage from a prominent 'post-structuralist' English-language commentator on French Theorists Gilles Deleuze and Pierre-Félix Guattari. It reads as a series of stipulative definitions, of 'the subject' etc., and is clearly (or fuzzily) a rewriting of some psychoanalytic ideas. But it mixes apparently empirical and therefore contingent propositions about bodies and 'subjects' with idiosyncratic definitional stipulations:

> The subject is the actualization of desire on the surface of bodies. It is in sense [sic] through an inscription of desire that bodies become subjects … Deleuze and Guattari make it clear that the problem of the subject is a problem of the 'subjectification' of desire, of inscribing breaks and flows of energy, joining and disjoining bodies (or partial bodies – the mouth, the breast, the anus, but also sounds and words and food, even the sun). The subject is not the body, but a composition (and effect) of bodies – a variable collection of organs, membranes, nerves and physiochemical processes, but also tools, means of nourishment and shelter and transport, the materials of production and consumption, etc. – a collection that somehow makes sense. ([sic] Bogard 1998: 67)

This sounds like a definitional paragraph. The author wants to stipulate that the word 'subject' will be used to refer to bodies causally related to their environments, and to others' bodies, perhaps. But it also sounds like a claim that 'the subject' is a newly 'discovered' entity, new to the way in which psychologists and sociologists think, at least. 'New' because, if you think of 'subjects' as William Bogard does, then you will learn something that you would not otherwise have known (in this case about the subjectification of people's bodies by society). A simple-minded reader might think they have learned something about actual babies becoming 'subjects' of society, and might even ask how this complex process works in relation to food or the sun. A naïve reader might worry about the use of 'etcetera' to avoid all the other possible factors that could be involved in 'subjectification'. But Theory is Theory, they might allow, not empirical description. Anyway, Bogard segues immediately to society:

> This is also the problem of society. Every society is a society of subjects fashioned from bodies, from an 'anorganic' plenum, from the assembly and disassembly of desiring-machines. Why 'machines'? Because this is literally [*sic*] what they are, assemblages that transfer, amplify or dissipate energy (but just as bodies must not be equated with organisms, machines must not be identified with inorganic, or non-living forms). Every sociology, from this point of view, is a sociology of desiring machines, and beyond that, of how those machineries are segmented and stratified, how bodies and their forces are distributed, coordinated, functionalized, and regimented to produce subjects. (Bogard 1998: 67–8)

This passage is also more stipulative than descriptive. Hence the proviso 'from this point of view', which implies that Bogard's general postulates and vocabulary be accepted as a precondition for making any empirical sense of the analysis. This is clear from what follows, which is literally an ecstatic pronouncement that the model of 'subjectivation' sketched in the earlier quote is part of a sociology of 'becoming – how to escape ... to dismantle rigid segments that individualize and bind the subject contingently to this body, this assemblage of bodies, these desires and habits'. So the writer returns to prosaic psychology, but now allows himself a Theoretical escape clause via the new-age promise of 'becoming'. (I shall consider the ubiquitous Cultural Studies notion of 'becoming' in detail in later chapters.)

Bogard uses Theory as a way of explaining more or less opposite outcomes at the sociological level. He asserts that 'the subject is always a matter of "*selection*"', which seems completely voluntary and free-willed, as he does not specify what or who does the selecting. On the other hand, 'it can be – potentially, virtually – a force of "absolute deterritorialization", of radical freedom, but also a force of the worst reaction and nihilism'. I will return to this apparently contradictory mix of romantic voluntarism and narrow determinism in later chapters. Here I want to acknowledge that, so far, I have been citing Theory as though it constituted one coherent body of conceptualizations and metaphysical assumptions. This is clearly an oversimplification. However, the Bogard example is typical of an increasingly popular way of writing about 'the subject' and sociology that Theorizes more or less everything in terms of a few concepts such as 'machines'.

'Cultural Studies' and/as Psychology

We might take 'culture' to mean something like *the shared and transacted meanings and values, the socially meaningful practices (including verbal, aesthetic, familial, sexual, etc.*

practices) of communities. In fact, the inchoate field that became known as 'Cultural Studies' began as a humanistic, anthropocentric but non-individualistic approach to studying the 'ways of life' of human communities (Williams 1981). Through the fertilization afforded by French literary semiotics (such as the writings of Roland Barthes) questions of what cultural practices and texts *meant* were foregrounded, as well as people's aesthetic responses to their own cultures. Meaning, shared and practised, passed on through generations, marked out as exclusive by sub-communities – these were the foci of typical Cultural Studies writing. This cross- or post-disciplinary field of academic writing began as a kind of anthropology of one's own culture(s).

As the examples I have quoted attest, however, Cultural Studies aspired to something grander than the study of culture(s) in the sense implied by my definition. Soon culture became a doorway into the anterooms of philosophical analysis that addressed issues of a methodological kind – questions that the humanities had addressed without embarrassment since the turn of the twentieth century: the nature of meaning; epistemology in the nonphysical 'sciences', indeed the very status of 'science' as a realist enterprise; the causes of cultural variation; the possibility of objective knowledge of something as mercurial as 'culture on the run' so to speak. Different cultures imply diverse human identities, differences that cannot be reduced to biological or psychological explanation based on the grand narratives of European post-Enlightenment thought (Darwin, Marx, Freud). Recently, Cultural Studies has implicitly challenged the assumptions of all schools of contemporary psychology, from evolutionary, bio/genetic theorizations of the causes of behaviour to behaviourist and cognitive approaches.

The post-disciplinary writing that emerged during the last third of the twentieth century questioned social sciences' claims to objectivity, promoting what might be called a cultural/political understanding rather than a deterministic, physical analysis of many psychological phenomena (including, most famously, 'schizophrenia' and 'racial' differences in measured IQ). A political celebration of 'difference' (especially sexual and ethnic 'difference') grew out of these re-theorizations of Anglo-American objectivism. Such a progressive and critical stance is not hard to understand. It must be remembered that during this period some influential psychologists had shown themselves to be happy to administer 'behaviour therapy' to try to change the sexual orientation of gay men and women, for instance, and that psychiatry (not to mention education) were deeply entwined with repressive social policy. By contrast, R.D. Laing in Britain and Thomas Szasz in the US proclaimed 'mental illness' a 'myth'. They argued for a cultural understanding of so-called psychological 'abnormality'. Indeed, they rejected normative models of psychological development and of mental 'health'. Instead, Laing saw schizophrenia as a 'problem of living' arising from extreme communication patterns within nuclear families, not as a physiological condition with specific symptoms. Guattari extolled the virtues of a method of radical critique of commonsense that he called 'schizoanalysis' (which today sounds very politically incorrect, given current knowledge about schizophrenia, but that is another story that I will not pursue here). Like Guattari, many French philosophers from the 1960s had proposed liberatory critiques of mainstream psychiatry, and of the West's 'liberal' political institutions, especially the family and the school, all of which they regarded as repressive, normalizing structures, or even as repressive 'machines'. The 'young Marx', Althusser, Freud and Lacan were in fashion. Then Barthes's and Foucault's socially relativistic discourse analyses redescribed popular culture high and low, marrying what Anglo-American academies had always seen as distinct realms of aesthetics and sociology.

Cultural Studies, as it came to be called in the Anglophone academies by the late 1970s, incorporated these new European enthusiasms into the analysis of culture and society. But, as it arose out of a rejection of social science and of 'high' cultural elitism (F.R. Leavis was a particular bête noire), its proponents became increasingly self-conscious about their own epistemological assumptions. Were they unreconstructed 'objectivists', 'realists', or 'humanists'? Should they embrace less-restrictive approaches to their study of cultural life and move beyond the boundaries and narrow methods of the older social and behavioural sciences? Cultural Studies academics who reached the midranges of their profession in the 1990s were educated in the 1960s and 1970s. They imbibed the radicalism sketched above as postgraduates or as young lecturers. They worked in Anglophone universities and watched the rigid disciplinary borders fall.

Today, Cultural Studies writing highlights the anthropological, the quotidian, and the constantly negotiated meanings and values that flow through the texts (conversations, media products, clothing, social practices, etc.) that make up the 'whole way of life' of people. It is 'post -', or perhaps, 'cross -' disciplinary, where the disciplines it critiques and revises include anthropology, literary studies, sociology. By the twenty-first century, Cultural Studies included dense, self-conscious Theorising about what it means to be human, about what humanism means, and thus became explicitly philosophical and psychological. For example, as we shall see in a later chapter, Cultural Studies writers speculate and theorize about the nature of human nature and its techno/cultural 'construction', and often do so in ways that cut across or deny the assumptions usually made in empirical psychology and in Western philosophy. The most egregious example of this, one that intrudes regularly into this book, is Brian Massumi's flag-waving Cultural Studies text, *Parables for the Virtual*. It begins where William James ended, a century or more earlier. Massumi sketches as background Leibnitz, Spinoza and Bergson, before modestly claiming that his way of dealing with a 'tumble of abstract intrigues' promises 'miraculous lucidity' though he admits it could become an uncontrolled 'black hole.' Whatever judgement a reader makes, his book offers nothing if not a radically new meta-psychology. It is Theory par excellence.

There can be no objection to this field of academic writing in principle, of course. Indeed, its ambition is laudable, however grandiose. Cultural Studies has:

- Sought to relativize and liberalize our understanding of concepts like 'race' and gender' identity
- Criticized as essentialist and pseudoscientific many concepts in psychology: 'personality', psychiatric 'illness', unidimensional intelligence, for example

- Drawn attention to the reification of many sociological and psychological concepts, and therefore to their conservative consequences
- Argued for an 'ecological', context-sensitive understanding of human cognition as relational, rather than accepting crude representationalist and mentalist approaches
- Opened up to analysis many social and sociopsychological practices by seeing them as *cultural* and not as 'natural' expressions of an essential humanity
- Investigated sociocultural phenomena of great diversity through richly-textured qualitative (e.g. semiotic, ethnomethodological) approaches
- Seen culture as implicated in all human behaviour, even that which is accepted as primarily physiologically determined, for instance schizophrenic 'symptomatology'

It must be admitted that Psychology had often presented only a narrowly empirical – some would say 'biologistic' or 'reductive' – and therefore limited account of its central concepts. However, Cultural Studies writers did not just take issue with the clinical, experimental, or historical evidence that is usually at stake within Psychology; they did not simply dispute the 'facts'. Rather, they questioned the status of 'facts' themselves. Instead of entering into debates about, say, the *nature and causes* of human psychological phenomena, identity or diversity, Cultural Studies reconceptualized the individual 'subject', many writers rejecting conventionally realist bio-psychological terms completely.

It is difficult to convey the detail of how the radical revision of conventional psychological concepts and assumptions (of causality, etc.) has been effected in the name of Cultural Studies. But let me illustrate this ambition by citing a passage from a book review in *Cultural Studies Review*, published in 2003.

> Colebrook then turns her attention to the role of perception in the 'noninterpretative' approach to life: 'Perception is used by Deleuze in its broadest possible sense, as a connection, interaction or encounter with the plane of life' (Colebrook, 2002, p. 140). Perception is an event grasped molecularly, but on a continuum right up to the human brain (the theatre in which actuality is screened) that slows down, delays and mediates perception, in the process forming assemblages (for example, faciality) and overcoming them (for example, the hand withdraws and becomes a tool) with the assistance of technical machines.
>
> The technical machine at issue here is cinema, which can be used to perceive perception through certain images of movement and time. Colebrook writes elegantly and insightfully on slowness in perception – slowing down perception introduces order. (Genosko, 2003: 227–28)

The most obvious difficulty here results from the attempt to postulate *a series of actual processes for which no empirical warrant is given, indeed for which none is even thought necessary*. Yet the passage discusses psychological matters: perception, tool use, the formation of mental concepts such as 'faciality', etc. How could the author or reader observe or infer 'perception slowing down', for instance, unless through elaborate experimental methods? The passage also begs many other psychological questions about which evidence is available: for example, is the perception of faces 'formed' (learned?) or does it also involve innate neurological circuits like 'mirror neurons', species specific mechanisms 'built into' actual brains? Most psychologists would regard this as an *empirical question*. It cannot be answered by means of introspection, however elegant the use of words to describe the phenomena that are claimed to be at issue. To accept this passage as writing about *real psychological phenomena* we would have to accept Deleuze's peculiar ontology that the author assumes. This includes (if we are to believe Colebrook and Genosko) accepting the following:

> Cultural Studies as it is practiced [*sic*] today has difficulty confronting immanence; immanence was a 'crucial idea' ... of Deleuze's philosophy. Cultural Studies needs, from a Deleuzian perspective, to be overcome or at least to learn to modify its reliance on representational thought and open itself to reinvention, becoming able to respond to the dynamically open flows and becomings of life, in all their speeds and durations and potentialities, beyond the human, which is 'just one type of imaging or perception among others'. (Genosko 2003: 277 citing Colebrook 2002).

Without analysing the passage in detail, it is clear that some prominent Cultural Studies writers see it as the task of their discipline to engage deeply with philosophical-psychological questions. Others, such as John Frow, see Cultural Studies as purely 'textual and 'intertextual':

> Cultural studies is a way of contextualising texts of any kind – of analysing the social relations of textuality; and there's no reason why it shouldn't include literary texts and literary regimes amongst its proper objects of knowledge ... It shifts the interpretive gaze from a self-contained text to its discursive and social framings, within which students are themselves implicated; while at the same time it opens up potentially fruitful methodological exchange between distinct protocols of interpretation that apply in the Social Sciences and textual disciplines. (Frow 2005)

To recontextualize texts of any kind, and to open up the 'fruitful methodological exchanges' recommended by John Frow, students are expected to display at least some (real or affected) knowledge of post-war continental philosophy, the critique of empirical sciences (both human and physical), Marxism, feminism, 'queer' theory, as well as the paradigms that they are assumed to have swept away (behaviourism, positivism, sociological functionalism, etc.). This is a tall order, even for accomplished academics that have immersed themselves in these fields for a decade or more. It is simply unrealistic, and more than a little insulting to undergraduates, for their academic mentors to pretend that they will be able to master the pros and cons of all these issues without being given the opportunity to study them directly within disciplines such as Philosophy, Linguistics, Psychology or Sociology.

Not surprisingly, Cultural Studies 'as she is taught' seldom rests on any precise knowledge of the disciplines its curricula consign to irrelevance. So one of its failures has been to misunderstand that science itself trades in interpretation as part of explanation, and that means '*theoretical* recontextualization'. There are not many vulgar 'science-as-facts' apologists still standing, in the social sciences especially. Yet this imaginary 'enemy' is the target of many recent metaphysical critiques that students are expected to accept. On the other hand, Cultural Studies has attempted to liberate students from dogma and from the sterile, trivial study of facts isolated from their social and cultural contexts. John Frow warns that Cultural Studies itself will not survive if it is 'taught as a form of religion', which is how he seems to see the status of many social science disciplines in the Western academy. So Cultural Studies is more a 'discursive domain' than a 'discipline' in the methodological sense, because it is defined by its textual 'ad hoc-ery' rather than by its commitment to *methodological* procedures. At the same time it is often metaphysically prescriptive, although, like many prescriptions, it is often illegible to all but the initiated.

Texts and Science

If Cultural Studies were merely a 'discursive domain', then so, some of its proponents assumed, were all academic disciplines. Hence the knowledge and theoretical vocabularies of science were just another 'discourse'. So scientific propositions could only be understood relative to the interests of those who proposed them; knowledge claims were made in the language of particular communities of experts and were not unmediated representations of 'reality'.

This view of science provoked acrimonious (and often amusing) debate. Notoriously, Alan Sokal and Jean Bricmont (1998) published an exhaustive critique of Theory's misappropriation (as they saw it) of the concepts and the assumptions about reality made by mainstream scientists. One of the French writers they enjoyed exposing as ignorant of the meaning and contexts of physical science concepts was Gilles Deleuze (whose influence on Cultural Studies is also discussed throughout this book). The debate continues. For instance, Australian Cultural Studies writers Andrew Milner and Jeffrey Browitt sought to defend Deleuze against Sokal and Bricmont's charges by distinguishing scientific from nonscientific discourse. They wrote:

> And they [Sokal and Bricmont] found Deleuze guilty ... of deploying valid technical terms in the service of argument 'devoid of both logic and sense' (p. 156). The nonsense is not always so obviously nonsensical, however; sometimes it is *simply non-scientific*. So, for example, when they take (prominent psychoanalyst Luce) Irigaray to task for her view that Einstein's $E=mc^2$ is masculinist for 'having privileged what goes the fastest', they miss the point that *the equation might indeed be masculinist even if it is experimentally verified* ... [T]he social genealogy of a proposition has no logical bearing on its truth value. (Milner & Browitt 2002: 100, 191, emphasis added)

Milner and Browitt defend Irigaray's interpretation or 'reading' by saying that it is 'political' rather than 'scientific': 'In short, Sokal and Bricmont simply disagree with Irigaray's version of radical feminist politics ... Politics and mysticism might often be, not so much opposed to science, as different from it' (Milner & Browitt 2002: 192).

I hope that readers will agree with me this is utterly tendentious: clearly, it is not with Irigaray's version of feminist politics that Sokal and Bricmont disagree, but with her version of the *meaning of the equation*. This is not merely a textual matter. Milner and Browitt's fairly typical counter-argument to Sokal and Bricmont is no argument at all. It avoids the point at issue and certainly does not justify as equally legitimate, ad hoc interpretations of physical science. It leaves open the question of whether *political interpretations* such as Irigaray's *can themselves be evaluated in terms of their truth or falsity*, even as they admit that it can be so judged by allowing that 'the equation might indeed be masculinist'. But are all 'interpretations' equally valid? I think not. It seems fair to see Irigaray's statement as 'nonsense' because it is epistemologically equivalent to saying that 'Newton's First Law of Motion is protestant', or 'Boyle's Law is pale blue'. If interpretation of scientific propositions is to include arbitrary recontextualizations that do not ask to be judged as true or false by any public means, then it seems fair not to treat them as intellectually serious.

If nothing else, this little contretemps is a reminder that Cultural Studies waded into the 'Science Wars' despite a distinct lack of appropriately-engineered weaponry. It is a mystery why, armed with no more than the linguistic slings and arrows of Theory, Cultural Studies writers felt they should fight epistemological (and indeed ontological) wars on the terrain of the *physical* sciences as well as in the territory once occupied by the *social* sciences. It is hardly surprising that humanities students ignorant of the Newton, Einstein or 'string theory' find themselves defenceless against *opinions* masquerading as *Theoretical propositions*.

Theory's Challenge

Humanities and the social sciences study the whole range of people's richly-diverse communicative practices, from graffiti emblems to racist 'science', from clothing and fashion to reality television programmes, from e-mails to *Macbeth*. Writing about such texts, their uses and 'meanings within context', involves revising many of the assumptions of empirical psychology. For Psychology has also been concerned with what, and how, people mean when they communicate. It has also sought to *explain*, to specify *the necessary and/or sufficient conditions* for precisely-defined, observable or inferable *behaviours*, experiences, human interactions, and so on. Simply put, Psychology assumes that the characteristics of the species, coupled with its particular interactions with biosocial reality, *cause* people to develop, interact and to behave as they do.

What is at stake in Cultural Studies' methodological/philosophical revisions of the goals of academic psychology? The following chapters address at least the following:

- The adequacy of current notions of 'life' and of biological species
- The concept of the 'post-human' and 'humanism'
- The concepts of the psychological 'subject' and human 'subjectivity'
- Relativist versus 'realist' and objectivist claims to knowledge in Psychology, and in other social sciences
- 'Essentialism' and reductionism in accounts of such traditionally contentious issues as race and gender
- The value of phenomenological analysis of cultural and psychological phenomena
- The viability of novel concepts, such as 'affect' and 'becoming', for analysing actual psychosocial, aesthetic, and 'political' phenomena

The essays in this book consider both the methodological adequacy and the educational significance of some or all of these intertwined issues. Although most of my references are as recent as the last decade, this period has not been chosen arbitrarily. It follows the reactions to Sokal's celebrated (and maligned) 1996 'hoax', and to its successor, Sokal and Bricmont's *Intellectual Impostures* in 1998 (above). The overlapping essays confront 'head-on' typical Theory-inspired psychological and philosophical writing that currently struts and frets its way across the post-disciplinary stage. Many of these textual performances I judge to signify nothing, while others seek to signify just about everything, in prose of befuddling density. Nevertheless, I attempt to draw out the implications of 'Theory-speak' for academic psychology and, indeed, for much of what might be called 'folk' psychology. While I do not wish to defend naïve 'commonsense' I do criticize uncommon nonsense where I find it.

My motivation is educational: I therefore present methodological strategies to enable students themselves to critically evaluate Theory where they find it. I do not consider the whole field of Cultural Studies. The following essays are partial in two senses: they do not purport to exhaust the field of Theory, and they are motivated by my commitment to realist epistemology. However, my examples are neither extreme nor marginal to the new field of interdisciplinary theorizing. I have chosen writing that is typical of the anti-empirical and hypocritical 'realisms' (e.g. 'hyper-realism') found in the sprawling cross-disciplinary literature. So, although the cases I examine are amongst the most flamboyant of Cultural Studies, they are educationally central to the claims of the new discipline.

Chapter 2

What is Theory About?

Theories pass, the frog remains.
                                   Jean Rostand

What I have labelled 'Theory with a capital-T' is impossible to summarize. So in this chapter I try to illustrate the ambition and scope of Theory by quoting writers who have been influential in recent Anglophone Cultural Studies. I hope that an account of what Theorists *do* will illustrate the ways in which they have challenged and tried to transcend realist social sciences' methodologies. By 'methodologies' I will mean, throughout this book, both the practical empirical methods of the sciences as well as their conventions of analysis, argument, theory construction and evaluation. But, a warning: readers will need to bear with me as I try to give a clear explanation of the often unconventional abstractions by means of which Cultural Studies challenges accepted method and theory in conventional Psychology and dismisses the founding assumptions of Anglo-American analytical philosophy.

Immaterial Foundations

Theory is about 'creating concepts, extracting precepts and generating affects at the same time as it makes us see new things'. Theory is built on the ruins of philosophy, although that does not prevent its practitioners from asserting that it 'should operate in the philosophical manner outlined by Deleuze'. To begin to understand Theory and its appeal to Cultural Studies writers, it must be accepted that 'bad' philosophy is limited to producing what Hainge disparages as mere 'commentary', and that, like 'science', it 'creates out of a system of coordinates, a referenced chaos that presents what appears to be a stable, fixed ontology' (Hainge, 2002: 285). An 'ontology' is a theory of what exists, what can be warranted as really existing, perhaps. So it is unsurprising that 'sciences' are concerned to present ontological arguments. What is surprising, however, is that academics writing on topics like experimental music (e.g. Hainge), body art, or even the appeal of Frank Sinatra's blue eyes (Massumi, 2002), should speculate about ontological questions and the limits of science. Why is it necessary to dismiss as 'bad philosophy' any struggle to analyse and to 'explicate existing phenomena'? Why the obsession to coin new words and invent concepts, to reveal novel realities, to 'see new things', as Hainge describes his goal?

Theory writers in Anglophone Cultural Studies continually return to this commitment to transcend analytic Western philosophy, with what Hainge disparages as its 'always comprehensible' ontology, its 'set of axiomatics', its 'fixed forms'. Rather, the Theory writer should create 'dynamic forms' that enter into 'becomings', for

> Cultural Studies has no ontology of its own, it is an expression which can only come into being through contact with the external source or text that it is transforming, a system that has no being in and of itself, that cannot be said to have a stable centre, and which cannot then be used as an agent of territorialization. (Hainge 2002: 287)

I will resist the temptation to analyse this in detail, but point out how such elusive definitions of the field can sound incoherent: here, for instance, Cultural Studies only exists as it is practised, it is asserted – it is an 'expression' which only comes into being as an effect on sources and texts. This way of speaking makes one wonder how this effect (this 'coming into being') could be achieved. The field of Cultural Studies is a shifting set of 'expressions' – the texts that result when some methodologies transform other texts. It is unclear how this could result in a new ontology and avoid 'axiomatics', however, unless this is only claimed in the trivial sense that would render Cultural Studies immune to all empirical evaluation and counter-argument because it asks for no inter-subjective agreement about its 'expressions'. All 'transformations' must be judged equally valid and revealing because no inter-subjectively-agreed criteria could be relevant to evaluating any new 'expression'.

On this kind of definition, Cultural Studies differs from all other methods of textual 'transformation' or hermeneutics. Its ambitions are unbounded, its methods untrammelled by such logical constraints as the avoidance of self-contradiction. Of course, my point would probably be dismissed as 'bad philosophy', as slavish adherence to 'axiomatics', as a mere quibble in the face of Theory's revolutionary challenge to social science. Indeed, Cultural Studies Theory writers sometimes explicitly pose just this challenge:

> It is difficult to overstate the scope of Deleuze and Guattari's challenge to social theory. What they propose is nothing less than a new ontology of the social, of social being, grounded in a philosophical ontology of Being as pure difference or becoming. Being, for Deleuze and Guattari, is that which differs from itself, in nature, always already, in itself, qualitatively different. (Bogard 1998: 53)

Just as it is difficult to overstate the scope of post-structuralist writing about 'the ontology of the social' and of social being, so too is it difficult to avoid being struck by the apparent incoherence of some of the metaphysics by which Theory mounts its case against 'old ontology'. 'Social being' seems not to involve any actual social *beings*, hence no beings who could 'be' socially, if we accept the above. So it comes as a relief to find that other Theorists allow that beings do 'exist'. They see Theory as focused on the actual *biological* 'body' or bodies, ignoring the fact that these seem to have been vaporized by the abstractions of their fellow Theorists. (See Chapters 6 and 7 for critiques of 'Body Theory'.)

Clearly, 'critical writing today' is worried about what were once philosophically basic questions – metaphysical questions. This chapter introduces my critique, mounted from a realist perspective, of what I see as the most egregious consequences of anti-realist neo-psychological analyses made through the playful 'invention of concepts' urged by prominent

Anglo-American (and Australian) followers of Deleuze's philosophy. Students of literary and Cultural Studies are frequently expected to incorporate into their disciplinary understanding a self-reflective awareness of the benefits of post-structuralist epistemological scepticism. This is made clear in the many recent books written for humanities undergraduates that canvass Francophone 'Theory', especially books directed at cultural, literary, and, indirectly, at psychology and sociology students. So, bemused undergraduates must try to understand what might be meant by propositions such as:

> Deleuze and those of his generation sought to conceptualise both difference and becoming, but a difference and becoming that would not be the becoming *of* some being. (Colebrook 2002: 3)

I want to confront this proposal 'head-on', so to speak – to interpret it literally. I see no alternative than to accept at face value Colebrook's claims regarding Deleuze et al. This revolutionary statement is central to the methodologies recommended in a book showing students of literature how to think in post-structuralist ways. Yet it proposes nothing less than a novel metaphysics – a novel ontology. I empathize with students who might be expected to evaluate this founding premise in a book on literary theory and, like them, accept that writers who proclaim such radical interventions into post-disciplinary academic analysis expect to be interpreted literally, or 'at their word', as is said in English. That is, I will try to engage with these authors in good faith, confronting what they assert with realist and empirical theory and observations from psychology, where this is relevant. That this old-fashioned method of evaluating theories and meta-theory is only rarely possible, however, results from the incoherence and idealism of much of what students are asked to accept, usually without any argumentative support, in the writing that I discuss.

After the 'Sokal Hoax'

As mentioned in Chapter 1, the 'Science Wars' centred on epistemological relativism. These debates ran parallel to what became known as the 'Theory Wars' in the Anglophone humanities. The 'Theory Wars' disputed the value of the grandiose metaphysical systems, concepts and metaphors of French humanities writing (Eagleton 1997; Franklin 2000; Hodge 1999). The most polemical writing in Cultural Studies responded to the angrily-debated hoax that physicist Alan Sokal aimed at the journal *Social Text* and its readers. This imbroglio occurred more than decade ago, but its parodied targets – post-structuralism, pseudo-physics, and metaphors whose epistemological status, said Sokal, was misunderstood by their proponents – refuse to go away. They continue to embellish much of the writing that goes under the name of Theory within interdisciplinary Cultural Studies in the first decade of the new millennium.

Following the hoax, in 1998 Sokal and Jean Bricmont published *Intellectual Impostures*, a detailed critique of (mainly French) non-science writers' allusions to the physical and biological sciences. In this extended work the authors studiously avoided satire and hoax alike. They did not analyse in detail the epistemologies implicit in the mainly French works that, in their view, travestied accepted scientific concepts. Instead they reproduced extended verbatim quotations that they saw as self-incriminating. These included passages from books by Deleuze, and books co-authored by Deleuze and Guattari. Sokal and Bricmont asserted that insofar as these quotations *arbitrarily* 'invoke[ed] terms and concepts from physics and mathematics', they offered no understanding of psychological, social, and political phenomena (Sokal & Bricmont 1998: 145). In a long introductory essay they objected to what they regarded as the French authors' epistemological relativism. However, I will not address that essay here but, instead, concentrate on issues of what I call 'creative ontology', especially as this issue relates to psychology and sociology.

During the past decade the unedifying arguments and name-calling that followed the Sokal Hoax have reverberated through the halls of Anglo-American academia. However, humanities writers have seldom thought self-critically about the implications of the hoax and its aftermath. In the Australian-born journal, *Continuum: A Journal of Media and Cultural Studies*, mathematician James Franklin (2000) crossed epistemological swords with linguist Bob Hodge (1999). The sarcastic tenor of this clash illustrates how passionately the respective methodological positions have been presented. In my view, Hodge defended a rather hypocritical version of social constructionism against Sokal and Franklin.

Hodge engaged in an elaborate rhetorical game to demonstrate that, in fact, no hoax had been perpetrated, 'and if there was [one], that it was not about postmodernism' (Hodge 1999: 268). Treating the original hoax as though it had been intended as a genuine contribution to Cultural Studies, he avoided any need to evaluate directly its epistemological and ontological implications.

Australia is a nation given to satirical attacks on pomposity, so it was no surprise that one university quickly developed a satirical *postmodern essay generator*, a device that, at the click of a cursor, produced neologistic essays suitable for undergraduate submission as postmodern assignments: a cornucopia of mini-Sokal Hoaxes! By contrast, the actual Humanities in Australia have continued as though the Sokal Hoax was no more than a rhetorical exercise – a social construct indeed – lacking implications for debates about how one might justify the claim to know things about an objective physical or social world.

So fiercely competitive has the university system become, and so insistent the demand for publications in refereed journals, that throughout the nineties the Humanities suffered from an oversupply of new doctoral graduates seeking academic employment. Interdisciplinary doctorates (from literature, fine art, film and media studies, etc.) were increasingly likely to be written in an explicitly 'post-structuralist' style: this often meant 'Deleuzian' if they derived from the Arts, and 'social constructionist' if they arose from what remained of the social sciences. The growth of Cultural Studies as a separate interdisciplinary field melding Literature, Sociology and Philosophy is itself evidence of these developments.

What is Theory About?

Ten years after the initial hoax, interdisciplinary fields of study in the 'post-disciplinary' humanities continue to reflect on their own epistemologies in ways that might strike Sokal and his physicist colleagues as logically confused or worse. For example, many writers in the 'new humanities' continue to assume that 'post-structuralist' epistemology has general implications for all fields of 'knowledge production' or 'practices', and many seem to characterize all conventionally-accepted scientific knowledge as illegitimate and naïvely 'objectivist'. Indeed, metaphors from physics and the howlers that infested the pseudoscientific writing that so amused Sokal continue into the new century, largely due to the influence of Deleuze and his Anglophone followers, such as the cross-disciplinary exegete, Brian Massumi (to whom I now turn).

Theory is Not Metaphor

This section of my enquiry into 'what Theory is about' is necessarily complex. So I ask for the reader's patience and assure her that the passages I am about to cite are intended to convey, in their own words, Theory-writers' ambition to revise completely Western psycho-philosophy. I will try to show that such a desire goes well beyond coining metaphors or figurative interpretations of psychological and aesthetic phenomena. Theory is meant to be taken literally – even Massumi's peculiar brand of psychology:

> The distinction between the living and the nonliving, the biological and the physical, is not the presence or absence of reflection, but its directness. Our brains and nervous systems effect the autonomization of relation, in an interval smaller than the smallest perceivable, even though the operation arises from perception and returns to it ... In all living things autonomization is effected by a centre of indetermination (a localized or organism-wide function of resolution that delinearises causality in order to relinearise it with a change of direction: from reception to reaction) ... At the fundamental physical level there is no such mediation ... The place of physical non-mediation [sic] between the virtual and the actual is explored by quantum mechanics. Just as higher functions are fed back – all the way to the subatomic (that is position and momentum) – quantum indeterminacy is fed forward. It rises through the fractal bifurcations leading to and between each of the superposed levels of reality. On each level, it appears in a unique mode adequate to that level. On the level of physical macrosystems analysed by Simendon, its mode is potential energy and the margin of 'play' it introduces into deterministic systems (epitomized by the three body problem so dear to chaos theory). On the biological level, it is the margin of undecidability accompanying every perception, which is one with a perception's transmissibility from one sense to another. On the human level, it is that same undecidability of every structure of ideas (as expressed, for example in Gödel's incompleteness theorem and in Derrida's *différence*. ([sic] Massumi 2002: 36–7)

This verbal torrent is intended to help the reader understand something – indeed, more or less everything, it would seem – about human 'life':

> Each individual and collective human level has its own peculiar 'quantum' mode; various forms of undecidability in logical and signifying systems are joined by emotion on the psychological level, resistance on the political level, the spectre of crisis-haunting capitalist economies, and so forth. These modes are fed back and fed forward into one another, echoes of each other one and all. (Massumi 2002: 37)

However, contrary to Sokal and Bricmont's generous criticism that this style of writing can be seen as largely *metaphorical*, recent Theory writers assert that it is not meant to be so interpreted:

> *The use of the concept of the quantum outside quantum mechanics, even as applied to human psychology, is not a metaphor.* For each level, it is necessary to find an operative concept for the indeterminacy that echoes what on the subatomic level goes by the name of quantum. (Massumi, 2002: 37, emphasis added)

This startling theorizing is made despite Massumi's equation of Derridean *différance* with Godel's theorem. Yet the passage can only be interpreted as referring to material reality – to quantum mechanics concepts being valid when adopted in psychological analysis (explanation?) as well as in sub-atomic physics. Neither reference is metaphorical, so they must be literal or denotative in intent. Similarly, earlier in his influential book Massumi had asserted that Deleuze postulates that 'ideality is a dimension of matter (also understood as encompassing the human, the artificial, and the invented)' ([*sic*] Massumi 2002: 36). Clearly, the writer not only assumes a novel kind of ontology, he also expects his readers to know of Gödel's theorem and Derrida's philosophy of language. So, even educationally, it is hard to justify this kind of writing. To understand it, the reader would need to be able to draw coherent implications from its propositions; in this case, to draw implications about the subatomic causes (?) of psychological phenomena, presumably.

A second example of a novel psychological ontology comes from a paper by Andrew Murphie, published in the prominent literary journal, the *Canadian Review of Comparative Literature*. This passage is also explicitly psychological and intended to be read literally, not metaphorically or analogically. It seems to be a piece of literally descriptive/explanatory metapsychology. It speaks of 'determinants', 'operations which form ...' etc:

> These two levels of perception, unconscious and conscious, though thoroughly interdependent, are quite different operations which form two heterogenous series. Yet there are no absolutes. What might provide a heterogenous series of minute perceptions for a cell of the body might provide a differential for a molecule in that cell. What provides a moment of perception for a muscle might be the result of a differential of many cells'

heterogeneous, minute perceptions ... What Deleuze, through Leibnitz, is suggesting here is that *all* perception is based upon this extraction of a clear zone of perception from fuzzy perceptions by a virtual differential. (Murphie 1997: 729)

Later in the same essay one comes across phrases such as '... bodies are intensifications of relations', glossed from Deleuze, who has written that 'intensity is the determinant in the process of actualization. It is intensity which dramatises' (Murphie 1997: 729).

Readers are entitled to assume that this passage conveys some denotative meaning. It seems to propose that something is the case, so to speak. However, it is difficult to know how to interpret the assertions made here because their ontological status is hedged about by low modality disclaimers ('might provide', 'might be the result', etc.). But this much is clear: if this way of writing is 'about' how people actually perceive the world, then we have a revolution in the human sciences under our noses and we should try to understand it. On the other hand, if Murphie is not making at least hypothetical claims about contingent phenomena that disciplines such as Psychology have traditionally sought to understand, then perhaps this is because, in the post-disciplinary world, knowledge is not what it used to be. And it is not what it used to be partly because, in such commentaries, abstract language takes precedence over communicating about reality: nouns are cobbled indiscriminately from verbs; adjectives, conventionally predicated of phenomena (to draw attention to aspects of them, so to speak), are used in grammatically idiosyncratic ways; relations are turned into nouns, and qualities attributed to them. How can one understand the proposition that 'bodies are intensifications of relations'? And what support could be advanced for the putative *description* of cellular, molecular and global levels of unconscious and conscious perception?

If nothing else, my cited example shows that, regardless of the Sokal Hoax, Anglophone Philosophy, Psychology and the life sciences are increasingly seen as fertile pre-texts for post-structuralist ontological claims. As recently as 2006, Murphie re-visited the question of the ontology of 'life' itself, again under the obvious influence of Deleuze and of Massumi. Analysing computer-mediated experience, he says of 'life and technics':

The proliferation of specific concepts of life is beginning to show that life is not ultimately to be defined, but is found instead in process, specificity and plurality; in the interstices ... It is found in the interstices even of those technical practices and ideas that are meant to capture and control life via tight procedures and narrow redefinitions. Life emerges from the interstices to extend performance management, or outmanoeuvre the intellectual property borders set up by biotechnology corporations. (Murphie 2006: 1)

Leaving aside the somewhat arbitrary examples in the last sentence, let me simply note that the passage's mode of confounding factual propositions with implicitly definitional stipulations is characteristic of much of the writing that was so savagely parodied by Sokal and exposed as incoherent by Sokal and Bricmont. Yet it persists, its authors doggedly committed to the practice of idealist reification and obfuscation, evident in terms like 'process', 'plurality' and 'interstices ... of ideas'.

Murphie's paper attempts, amongst other things, to redefine what it means to attribute 'life' to phenomena, but seems to argue that 'life' is *relational* – that it is not a quality, aspect or characteristic of organic entities. Hence, it implies, Cultural and Media Studies need to reconceptualize understandings of mediated interactions between people and their life-worlds/technics, etc. in more dynamic ways (recall Colebrook's use of 'becoming' as a noun, earlier). But Murphie assumes both an ontology and an epistemology that make little precise sense other than as metaphors or rhetorical pleas for a less positivistic approach to the issues he discusses. Obviously, this kind of writing is a response to the challenge to understand the digital/virtual *mediation* of much of contemporary social and mental life. And one can detect an attempt to propose that *relations* between and amongst humans (although he might baulk at the term) and their respective, ever-changing environments (technologies, tools, etc.) must be thought of as *interactive*. So he cites Whitehead, who asserts that 'occasions of experience are the really real things, which in their collective unity compose the universe' (Murphie 2006: 10). For Murphie, this is 'not abstraction or idealism', a position which is consistent with his notion that '[t]here is no "essential" body as against technics' (Murphie 2006: 6). This seems to mean that bodies cannot be described – cannot be attributed qualities – without regard to their actual or possible environments of adaptive support. Bodies cannot, in fact, exist in isolation. But, surely, this is an empirical matter; it does not imply that bodies cannot be conceptualized in isolation and some of their qualities described.

The root cause of these confusions is the failure to distinguish between attributing qualities to objects (e.g. the ability to metabolize fuel/energy that seems a necessary condition for the claim that something qualifies as 'alive') and the implications of treating such objects as, in fact, capable of surviving in isolation. Murphie wants to avoid 'essentialism'. That is, he is at pains not to attribute fixed, invariant qualities to objects for fear of violating a Deleuzian tenet that prioritizes 'becomings' over 'dumb' material things.

The socio-technological contexts to which Cultural Studies writers are responding are difficult to describe briefly. They include the rapid commercialization of digital technologies; cybernetics; the cultural exploration of virtual worlds; the revolution in molecular biology (especially genetics); not to mention hyper-consumerism and increasing 'globalization'. Predictably, these developments have been addressed frequently from the perspective of Cultural Studies 'Theory' rather than sociologically. Typically, in the paper I have quoted, Murphie brings together biological and technological developments. He employs the language of 'emergence' to move beyond what Cultural Studies sees as banal physical and biological knowledge of 'dumb matter'. I shall return to this kind of writing when I discuss 'vitalism' in Chapter 6.

Deleuze-inspired strands of Theory deal with several weighty problems. These include problems of language and its relationship to the 'outside/real' (and 'inside/ mental') worlds; the so-called virtual world of cyberspace; human experience and subjectivity; scepticism about semiotic processes and chaos theory as a metaphor for global complexity and uncertainty. To follow Deleuze is to invent concepts intended to displace earlier psychological and political-sociological paradigms that became consolidated during the 1960s and 1970s. But notwithstanding the epistemological caution that the Sokal Hoax could have encouraged, many of the assumed foundations of the humanities and of biopsychology have been rewritten as ecstatically abstract 'Theory' during the past decade.

Indeed, the examples I have cited are unusual only in their *explicitly* idealist approach, which sees *definition alone* as constitutive of knowledge. Typically, 'Theory' writers simply assume that empirico-realist epistemologies are passé. Sokal's embarrassing intervention has not slowed the proliferation of ontological speculation that it most blatantly exposed to ridicule. Ironically, as the detailed analyses I will present in Chapters 3 to 7 attest, the implications of the hoax have been largely avoided by shifting the debate away from epistemology towards ontology. I will argue that this has only compounded the problems that face potential humanities and social science students. Both Sokal's Hoax and Sokal and Bricmont's provocative book concentrated on the peculiar ignorance and grandiose claims made, largely *en passant*, about the physical sciences by 'poststructuralist' writers. My focus is narrower: as this chapter has begun to do, I will concentrate on what happens when Theory is employed ostensibly to clarify psychological, philosophical and sociological questions. I am particularly concerned with the *educational* implications of these unconventional and highly ambitious revisions of older academic disciplines.

Chapter 3

Different Things

Things ain't what they used to be.
                                          Ted Persons

Language Problems

Some of the motivation for Cultural Studies' rejection of mainstream academic psychology is easy to understand, indeed to sympathize with. It is hard to deny that many sub-fields of post-war Anglo-American Psychology have become increasingly atomized into cells of narrowly-specialized research-generated research. Accumulating micro-facts while ignoring questions of what gives lives meaning and how people negotiate their respective narratives, academic psychology has narrowed its vision, leaving to literature, including journalism and popular culture, the task of trying to understand the complexities of lived experience, pleasure and suffering. Humanities students will search Psychology curricula in vain for analyses of people understood holistically as social beings enmeshed in culturally-rich histories. Psychology textbooks seldom convey any sense of the struggles of lives lived in difficult circumstances, let alone the 'unfolding-ness' of individual biographies or of resonant human sub-cultures.

Cultural Studies has sought to convey the textures of lived lives, the complexities and subtleties of linguistic and other cultural systems and their use. Unlike cultural anthropology and cultural psychology, it has turned away from objective accounts of comparative cultural phenomena, moved away from explanation towards interpretation and tried to convey the phenomenology (such as the narrative and emotional significance) of 'otherness', for example. Instead of explaining why cultures are different objectively, Cultural Studies assumed that social and cultural 'science' was an unnecessary, indeed impossible, enterprise. To turn cultures into 'things' and to pretend to study them 'objectively' – to explain them 'scientifically' – was metaphysically mistaken and ethically indefensible.

Many Cultural Studies writers have gone further. Much of the discipline accepts as unarguable the view that the way language was used in the social and psychological disciplines was both epistemologically untenable and ontologically limiting. Contrary to commonsense views, it was argued that words cannot simply represent things (situations or events included); no adequate or complete description of events and entities is ever possible; language is not a reliable communicational medium; language is neither objectively analysable, nor objectively 'useable'. The view that culture and society could be studied as though language was 'transparent', as though it mirrored, or corresponded to, reality, was naïve. It led to scientism (the idea that human cultures and social life could be explained objectively on the model provided by physical science).

It is true that how language is used in all science is philosophically problematic. But because science is a public, contestable practice, scientific method demands clear and, as far as possible, unambiguous communication. This means that scientists are obliged to take great pains to present to their readers *explicitly defined concepts*. They must take care to avoid ambiguity and equivocation so that the whole community of scientists working on the one set of problems knows that it is speaking 'the same language' about 'the same thing'. Inter-subjective reliability is encouraged by explicit definition of 'low level' (observable) and 'higher level' (abstract) concepts alike.

Cultural Studies, however, is not only suspicious of the possibility of unambiguous concepts but also generally reluctant to define its terms in ways that would allow its practitioners to be confident that they are speaking about the same (class of) phenomena. It is more than a little ironic that Cultural Studies scepticism about the possibility of linguistic reference is often given as an argument against those who try to use language unambiguously to refer to actual phenomena (including complex and abstract ideas). Ironic, because scientists' careful definitional practices might dissolve many of the apparently complex metaphysical and methodological paradoxes that cultural Theory stumbles over, especially as these relate to actual humans and their psychology.

A dominant theme running through my attempts to untie the various conceptual knots of Theory as they relate to psychological matters centres on the use of language and the need for clear definition of terminology. This I also see as an ethical issue. It is unfair to one's reader not to define as unambiguously as possible the terms of one's analysis or argument. Similarly, one should not assume that the provenance or conceptual context of one's vocabulary is common knowledge, especially amongst undergraduates. In the following chapters, therefore, I return to the question of how and whether concepts are defined within their respective theoretical contexts. More than once I make the point that, especially in post-disciplinary textbooks, radical scepticism about the communicative effectiveness of language sits uneasily beside grandiose metaphysical and pseudo-scientific writing, the principal function of which is to exploit for no more than literary effect the very ambiguity that could be avoided by the simple expedient of explicit definition. By contrast, I remain sceptical not of language as a mode of communication but of Theory writers' proposed solutions to the problems of understanding cultural life and lives through language. I want to reassure students that the propositions of modern psychological science (the explanatory accounts of what causes people to behave and to communicate in particular ways) are usually meaningful, contestable public statements like any others that refer to objective reality. So too are those labelled Cultural Studies when they offer different theoretical accounts of what is the case. All may be judged false or ambiguous, vague or trivial, of course, but making just such judgements is the point of a methodologically sophisticated education.

This chapter deals with several interrelated issues around how psychologists and cultural studies writers use and define language. I consider methodological concepts that loom large in criticisms of commonly-accepted explanations of socio-cultural phenomena – 'reductionism' and 'essentialism'. I then discuss two linguistic paradoxes that ensnare non-realist theory:

the term 'difference' and the problem of 'reification' of relations between and amongst phenomena. To conclude, I describe 'race' and 'ethnicity', and try to show that careful definitions can resolve many of the apparently complex methodological issues in which these terms are enmeshed, both in everyday conversation and in 'scientific' discourse. As will be apparent already, my approach is necessarily somewhat 'technical'. I make no apology for this: to understand and criticize the methodological revolution called 'Theory' demands subtle analytical stratagems. I propose several of these to enable students to evaluate the cogency of the literature currently named Cultural Studies, especially insofar as it proposes a peculiar view of the relationships that obtain between language and the world.

Reductionism and 'Essentialism'

A central tenet of post-disciplinary critiques of social science accounts of culture is that they *reduce* complex phenomena to single, fixed categories. They petrify *(reify)* linguistic terms and reduce to fixed categories the complex dynamics of ever-changing 'life' and the infinite variety or differences amongst things. Because classification is essential to explanation, this may result in narrow, spuriously 'objectivist' claims to have 'explained' complex social or cultural phenomena.

Cultural Studies writers argue against naïve and limiting psychological concepts that are all too frequently invoked to 'explain' phenomena such as sex roles and ethnic differences. Cultural theorists refuse to see these as *exclusively biologically determined*. Instead, cultural writers regard biological factors as irrelevant to understanding the significance of gender identity and or ethnic difference. Their critique of Psychology finds a large target in neo-Darwinian accounts of various social and cultural phenomena couched in the language of genetic determinism or 'evolution'. Examples of reductionist analyses are easy to find in contemporary academic psychology and in popular versions of its central concerns. The much-published popularizer of psychology, Stephen Pinker, recently presented an analysis of human morality that linked it to biological evolution. He wrote that, by analogy with Chomsky's 'universal grammar for language', 'we are born with a universal moral grammar that forces us to analyse human action in terms of its moral structure, with just as little awareness') as we have of grammatical structure (Pinker 2008: 26).

It will come as no surprise to learn that Cultural Studies writers see this kind of biological reductionism as simplistic. Pinker implies that cultural diversity and change are not created through human cultural forces. Ethical systems are 'reducible' to the biologically effective; they are fated to evolutionary inevitability. Pinker defends the claim that 'the moral sense is an innate part of human nature' by saying that this is 'not far-fetched'. But he excludes cultural-historical interpretations of complex human behaviours and social institutions (such as those that dispense justice, for instance). This is an egregiously 'reductionist' argument as it stands, although, to be fair to Pinker, he does try to avoid the narrowest implications of his postulates, and allow a more open possibility:

> Perhaps we are born with a rudimentary moral sense and as soon as we build on it with moral reasoning, the nature of moral reality forces us to some conclusions and not others. This idea is called moral realism. (Pinker 2008: 27).

Obvious counterexamples to the notion of an evolution-based universal morality are easy to find. For example, it is tempting just to say that Pinker has obviously not met my two-year-old granddaughter or he'd be less sanguine about even a 'rudimentary' 'innate moral sense'! However, Cultural Studies has not generally countered reductive proposals with the empirical evidence of counterexamples. Instead it has argued that all scientific argument/explanation/analysis is based on *metaphysically* untenable, illusory 'foundations', as discussed in Chapters 1 and 2. Theory writers may question whether cause-and-effect relationships between discrete observable phenomena can be asserted at all. They may claim that only 'processes', 'becomings' and change can be postulated as ontologically 'foundational' (Colebrook 2002) and therefore that all universalistic explanation of what humans 'do' is simply naïve. In short, Theory's rejection of 'reductionism' is usually total; it goes well beyond that advanced within even philosophically-sophisticated psychology or biology.

Cultural Studies Theory sees what it calls 'essentialism' as a version of reductionism. Essentialism involves attributing invariant or constant qualities to classes of objects. Such qualities, it is asserted, define and explain some of the behaviours exhibited by these 'objects' merely on the grounds that they are members of a particular class. 'Male/female' will serve as an obvious example of an essentializing binary construct in popular discourse. Essentialism is epitomized in the claim that '(sexual) anatomy is destiny' (attributed usually to Freud). To attribute *causal* sufficiency to a person's genes, and to essentialize 'gender' or 'race', would also be judged reductionist by most psychologists, of course. Similarly, any analysis could be regarded as essentialist if it argued that members of a particular class exhibited common qualities simply *by virtue of their membership of that class*. Racial categorizing and stereotyping commit this fallacy. Many psychologists have long been critical of such trivial or circular pseudo-explanation, but Theory writers extend the concept of essentialism to many fields of analysis beyond those usually considered by academic psychology (as will be seen in various contexts throughout this volume).

The blanket rejection of essentialism and reductionism in Theory, however, may lead writers into methodological cul-de-sacs. Despite their best intentions, some writers take the least elegant, certainly the least realist, route to analysing bio-psychological phenomena. Andrew Murphie and John Potts speak of 'life' as 'relational'; they ask that the concept not be reduced to the list of empirical qualities of a class of objects (that would be to postulate and essentialize what Massumi calls 'dumb matter'). Their relational approach to biological concepts is consistent with the analysis proposed by many philosophers of biology such as Stephen Rose. Rose criticizes 'reducing' (his word also) 'phenotypes' (actual biological beings) to their genes. He endorses instead the view that '[g]enes and environment are dialectically interdependent throughout any individual's lifeline'. For

Rose, the argument for genetic 'primacy' involves 'a reversion to an almost prescientific doctrine of preformation which we can surely now transcend' (Rose 2005: 133).

Rose cites the cultural-historical differences between attitudes to handgun ownership in Europe and the United States as a *non*-reductionist explanation of different levels of violence in the two societies: 'unlike reductionist ones, such hypotheses may provide pointers for meaningful intervention' (2005: 298). Obviously, cultural factors also point away from biologically essentialist explanations that would see different rates of violence between ethnic groups as expressions of 'racial' (genetically-determined) characteristics. Rose's objections to reductionism (and to essentialism) are in no way problematic. So it is easy to understand Cultural Studies' shared antagonism to such methodologically naïve social 'science'. It is clearly important not to reduce cultural and psychological – nor biological phenomena, for that matter – to invariant, physical 'essences' and thereby to postulate convenient, all-purpose 'causes'. Interestingly, in rejecting the physical reduction of biological phenomena, Rose uses the term of which Theory has become very fond: 'becoming'. For the biological theorist the word emphasizes the importance of dialectical 'process' over reified and static 'being'. However, he sensibly avoids the transcendental abstractions of much of what I call 'Theory' in this book. Unlike Colebrook, for instance, Rose is content to employ nouns to refer to actual objects, and verbs to designate real (including dialectical) processes and relations between actual phenomena.

Relations and Things

In the humanities, especially in literary fields, but even in political and legal studies, linguistic 'deconstruction' had been a fashionable methodological practice throughout the 1970s and 1980s, although few English-language analysts seemed to accept the radical implications of Derrida's scepticism for writing and communicating about a world that exists independently of language. That is, few recognized that 'deconstruction' presupposed meta-theories of language that contradicted most of the assumptions they themselves routinely made about language and representation in their less self-reflexive moments. In the new century, students of Cultural Studies are still frequently expected to accept *both* Derrida's 'anti-meaning' analyses as well as Deleuze's sometimes hysterical creation of concepts (or words at least) that propose a kind of alternative ontology (to which I have already alluded). Todd May (1997) considers both these theorists' use of the term 'difference' in his philosophical discussion of their respective works. However, he stops short of examining whether their radical paradigms are *logically compatible* with each other at any precise level of analysis. If they were not logically consistent with each other, of course, students could not be expected to assume the validity or usefulness, let alone the truth, of *both* deconstruction and Deleuze's ontological postulations. They could not, in good faith, trade on the different senses of one term, say 'difference', and use them interchangeably in their own university essays or theses. Nevertheless, many academics teaching Cultural Studies do appear to accept just such logical duplicity. They seem happily to accept *any* of Theory's postulates and practices, however self-contradictory, as long as these are antagonistic to the same 'enemies', namely 'realism', 'empiricism', 'positivism' – in short, all claims to objective knowledge made by Theory's bête noire, social and physical science.

Derrida has been subjected to intense analysis by at least some Anglophone critics. Robert Grant's brilliant, if intemperate, critique summarizes what he sees as Derrida's two principal poststructuralist errors:

> One is to suppose that conventional designations cannot genuinely refer. They can and do ... so long as we agree on what they refer to ... The other, closely related, error is to suppose that the only 'real' reference could be to a 'thing-in-itself', that is, to 'ultimate' reality. (Grant 1996: 275–6)

But, Grant stresses, to the contrary, that 'the only reference we have or need is to "things in their relation to man"' (1996: 276).

As we shall see, Deleuze sought to write about 'ultimate reality' without reference to actual people, and to pay lip service to Derridean scepticism about the referentiality of language use. This high-wire act is summarized by the philosopher of literature, Colebrook:

> The problem with appealing to experience, for Deleuze, was that we tend to assume some normative or standard model of experience, such as human experience of an outside world. (We have to ignore inhuman [*sic*] experience, such as the experience of animals, nonorganic life and even future experiences of which we have no current image). The problem of basing knowledge on structures was that any attempt to describe such a structure would have to pretend to be outside or above such structures ... If we want to understand the structure of our language we will have to use some sort of language to explain it. Even the term 'language' already relies on a structure of distinctions: we can imagine a culture that has no general term for language but might refer to 'signs' or 'symbols'. Deleuze's great problem and contribution was his insistence, in opposition to structuralism, on difference and becoming. (Colebrook 2002: 2)

Similarly, as I will discuss later, Massumi (2002) attacks not only what he and his followers see as the linguistic 'petrifications' and reifications of Western metaphysics, including the 'human subject' itself, but also the conceptual bases of empirico-realist epistemologies in general. Post-structuralist Theory is nothing if not ambitious! Massumi celebrates Deleuze's revolutionary metaphysics as an escape from all that is taken for granted in common (human) sense: cause-and-effect relations; linguistic referentiality; even, as suggested above, the very material 'stuff and objects' which students naïve enough to call themselves 'realists' think help to constitute 'the real' – all are reconceptualized by Theorists. The individual human is not seen as real in conventional ways: it is neither an agent nor an effect of social events, but instead is a node on a dynamic, horizontally-conceptualized network or plane of ever-changing abstract relationships. These are planes of 'impersonal [sic] affect and/or virtuality'. If my (necessarily brief) summary below, is fair, it leads to the conclusion that the Deleuzian ontology incorporated by Massumi into disciplines that were once called 'Aesthetics', 'Psychology' and 'Sociology', is so unconventional as to be difficult for the uninitiated reader even to imagine. However, in this chapter, I only want to draw attention to the problematic issue of how we use words to refer to abstract phenomena, and to highlight the possibility that a realist account can be advanced for many of the problems that Cultural Studies writers deal with as social or linguistic 'constructs'.

Becoming Theoretical

Fiona Hibberd (2005) reminds us that coherent discourse presupposes that knowledge of situations is possible and that 'situations are propositional in form'. Moreover, as she points out, realism need not posit a transcendental subject, reify relations, nor deny that the world is constantly in flux (all Deleuzian preoccupations, as will be seen). Ironically, the Theory writers whom I have cited have tried to *avoid* reification, so have proposed the 'non-foundational foundations' I considered in Chapter 1.

Deleuze and his followers reject the tenet that knowledge claims must be 'propositional'. This results from denying that the grammatical subject must be, to adopt Hibberd's phrase, a 'location of a predicated description'. It refers to an *entity with qualities that can be verbally designated*. For Deleuzians, such a notion is naïve (essentialist indeed!). It leads to a kind of petrification of static entities rather than to the preferred ontology of 'becomings'. However, I would argue that this claim itself involves mistakenly reifying a relation (i.e. 'becoming'), by proposing that a relation can *exist independently* of its relata; that is, by thinking relations are 'things', as I considered above.

'Becoming' derives from 'to become', and in English this is a transitive verb. So real situations in the world cannot coherently be said to consist of 'becomings' any more than they can of 'be-goings', or of 'larger-thans'. These are all *relational* terms. Of course, the universe is constantly in flux, but that may be irrelevant to the point at issue. Those who follow Deleuze down the path of 'becomings as entities' or as events quickly find that what exists remains ambiguous at key places in his analyses. For instance, discussing the infinitive he writes:

> The infinitive – 'to think', 'to green' [sic], 'to act', 'to write', 'to be' – does not admit of a division between what something is and what it does. There is the event itself and not some prior transcendence of which the event would be an act. (Deleuze 1990: 221)

Of course, the infinitive does not, by itself, imply that there is a transcendent 'subject' of which verbs are predicated. But nor do infinitives, as infinitives, *refer* to 'events' in most people's understanding of language. If infinitives could meaningfully be used to designate some kind of event, then Deleuze might well claim that the subject is not even a *discursive* necessity. But this is surely confused and leads to incoherence. He claims to want to avoid transcendental idealism. He tries to find some way of writing about things of which predications can be made that does not require him to postulate a 'transcendental' subject. But why is the subject thought of as 'transcendental' here at all, unless to beg the question at issue?

Colebrook pursues this odd argument in a slightly different way: for her, the subject is not 'denied' but seen as a 'virtual effect' (which some might regard as a subtle kind of denial anyway). She writes, 'For Deleuze, the reactivism of the subject is overcome not by denying the subject – but by affirming the subject as a virtual effect, and then by multiplying movements of subjective 'virtuality' (Colebrook 2002: 131).

I take this to mean that subjects (meaning subjective aspects of real people, not just *grammatical* subjects) must be only 'virtual' because they are 'effects' of something else. As used here, I suspect, 'virtual' means something like 'potential'. Still, this seems a dubious move: if the linguistic subject cannot be used coherently then calling it a 'virtual effect' still does not allow one to refer to any particular material phenomenon/a of which predication could be proposed. But then, in the Deleuzian universe, events seem to happen *without* any actual location; they happen 'to' no-one or no-thing in particular. This strikes me as a peculiar way of avoiding the 'transcendental metaphysics' that Deleuzians think bedevils Western Philosophy. Note that the 'virtual' is intended to extricate the proponent from the realist implications of his approach. On the contrary, however, it can be seen as leading to very odd metaphysics indeed. So it comes as no surprise to find commentators glossing 'the virtual' in an elusive but tautological way as 'potential for actualization' and postulating a potential infinity of such actualizations. This hardly seems to avoid idealist metaphysics.

What is called 'the virtual' in this kind of writing appears to offer only a verbal solution to Deleuze's problem. Indeed it confounds his epistemological dilemma, especially when he claims, according to his follower Colebrook, that

> [t]here is not a domain of the real that is … given to the subject. There is simply givenness, and the giving of the given cannot be located in the subject [sic] … It is not as though there is a real world (realism) that is repeated virtually in the subject (as ideal). The actual is a constant becoming virtual. (Colebrook 1999: 131)

So now the actual becomes virtual, but (above) the virtual also referred to potential for 'becoming actual'! A generous way of interpreting this obscure circularity might be to say that it seeks to avoid collapsing the relations designated by verbs into the entities designated by nouns (an aim which is also consistent with realism). The last Colebrook sentence above might mean something like, 'The real is always becoming *known*'. But, what is one to make of the proposition that 'there is simply givenness'? (Perhaps this should have been, 'Givenness is simply all that is given' (although we might have asked, 'to whom?' because 'to give' is a relational term itself!).

The distinction in English between transitive and intransitive verbs is not acknowledged in translations of French Theory, apparently. Hence brain-numbing locutions abound in which relations hold or obtain between no actual termini, and verbal processes occur without even grammatical subjects, let alone actual agents being nominated.

Relations are reified as 'things' and used as metaphysical conveniences in this discussion of philosophy's relevance to literary studies. The only purpose served by such tortuous abstractions, however, seems to be to avoid the charge that one believes that actual subject-predicate relations are epistemologically and ontologically 'foundational'. Why students would need to endorse this anti-foundational foundation in order to read Shakespeare or discuss *Bladerunner* is at best unclear. At worst, the recommended 'process ontologies' of Colebrook's version of Deleuze pointlessly befuddle and intimidate those they are intended to enlighten.

Real Differences? 'Race' and Identity

Nowhere is essentialism more common yet unnoticed than when race membership is attributed to individuals ('Barak Obama is the first "Black" president') or when psychological or physical qualities are attributed to so-called races (the labels for which are arbitrary, overlapping, and usually based on skin-colour). Race is assumed to be a quality of individuals, and membership of race(s) thought to be the logical equivalent of membership of of a club or family. But race is a tricky concept, and its use in academic and popular discourse frequently 'essentialist' and reductionist because people fail to understand that it is socially constructed and its use is not referential in a simple way.

'Race' is generally understood today as a social construct, a concept that emerged with the expansion of bureaucratic colonialism as an alibi for class and gendered oppression and exploitation (e.g. Dyer 1997). So it is not surprising that when 'scientific' empirical claims involving so-called races are asserted (such as hypothesized differences in some measurable psychological quality) they are routinely criticized as 'essentialist' and/or as 'positivist'. That 'race' is a social construct and that the term merely refers to 'differences' between and amongst people seem unarguable. It follows that 'races' are not actual biological phenomena; that is, so-called 'races' are not 'essentially' different (different 'in fact', or 'in reality', as is commonly said). Hypothetical 'racial differences' and therefore races, understood as *groups of people exhibiting different qualities or characteristics*, can be dismissed as ideological mystifications.

Given the emphasis on culture and semiotics that ground their work, few Cultural Studies writers would accept that race is an empirical concept, and therefore that it allows meaningful ways of classifying individuals into biologically-distinguishable groups. This naïve notion of 'race' has been displaced by a linguistic-cultural concept of 'ethnicity' rather than biologically-definable race. Cultures give meaning to race labels and to the concept itself. Some differences and not others are marked for *political* purposes (Barker 1999).

Ethnicity is not understood as based on physical qualities of persons or groups, but is a matter of subjective identification with labels, values, practices – with cultural definitions and descriptions.

A social scientific research project that is founded on this cultural and self-identifying notion of ethnicity, although still called 'race', was conducted by Darnell Hunt. He examined the ways by which differently 'raced' Americans (i.e. people who identified themselves under different classifications based on national-ethnic origins, and/or on skin colour) interpreted and evaluated television news representations of the 1992 Los Angeles 'race riots'. Hunt defined race (or 'race', at least) in subjective terms:

> In the contemporary United States, 'race' defines particularly salient subjectivities, locations from which actors construct and/or receive media texts and make sense of the world. At the same time what it means to belong to a race is continuously created intertextually. (Hunt 1997: 18)

That is, by means of various regimes of representation in US culture (in education, national political discourse, TV news reports, etc.).

A stronger version of race categorization as principally or entirely a matter of subjective identification has emerged in tandem with a generally social constructionist epistemological analysis of all biological and scientific concepts. Social constructionist accounts of race as an exclusively discursive concept see all race categorizations as complicit with empiricism and therefore as epistemologically naïve (a typical and influential example is Wetherell & Potter 1992.) In this view, race-mentioning statements are merely rhetorical, and can make no meaningful claims about biosocial reality. The role of critical analysis, then, is to 'examin(e) the discursive process by which true and false statements become distinguished' (socially), and not to endorse some statements as true and to reject others as false. Presumably this is because statements can only be *intra*-discursively meaningful, and cannot *refer to*, certainly not *represent*, extra-discusive reality – states of affairs, historical processes, biological qualities of individuals or groups, etc. So, as Wetherell and Potter argue:

> One of the main difficulties with what we are calling representational analyses of racist discourse – the analysis found in some accounts of ideology and in most social cognition research – is that what is assumed to be true becomes in some sense non-social, beyond investigation, while falsity or error become open to study and are seen as quintessentially social phenomena ... social influences are only brought in when some negative action, or some piece of error or 'misrepresentation' needs to be explained. (Wetherell & Potter 1992: 67)

On their terms, it is pointless to criticize racist beliefs as false or conceptually simplistic because the question of empirical truth is irrelevant to the force of racist discourse. This seems to follow from the assumption that empirical claims that invoke the concept of 'race' are *always and only* a matter of 'representation'. This point might be made differently by saying that Wetherell and Potter assume that propositions that include race concepts do not refer to real phenomena but to linguistic or semiotic practices only. So they reject critique from a realist epistemological perspective because

> This treatment of racist discourse, and this analysis of ideology, begin by defining ideological statements as inaccurate and misleading representations of reality. The possibility of an epistemological break between reality and appearance, truth and falsity or essential forms and phenomenal forms is thus raised ... One class of discourse, (the scientific), is thus privileged and its neutrality assumed in order to reveal the non-neutral and interested nature of other forms of discourse. (Wetherell & Potter 1992: 18)

Race terminology is, obviously, 'socially constructed'. But that may not mean that all knowledge claims invoking race categorizations are merely claims about the ways in which language is used. The question of the truth or falsity of racist (or, for that matter, non-racist) statements is independent of the social determination of how words are used. Social constructionism is an unhelpful epistemology insofar as it begs the question of the meaning of 'race' and of statements referring to or 'representing' biological and social phenomena in various contexts. This is because it assumes that all uses of the term are non-referring: race labels cannot in principle, as it were, designate situations, phenomena, 'things'. It allows for no way of preferring some contextually-specific uses of race categories over others. If all race concepts are equally unable to be deployed in empirically-contingent propositions, *by definition*, then we must presume that no true or false propositions can be relevant to the discussion of race, racism or race-as-representation itself.

Chris Barker exemplifies the contradictions in which much of Cultural Studies semiotic constructionist discussion of race quickly becomes ensnared. Rejecting the value of 'positive images' of 'black people' (he also happily speaks of 'white people'), Barker asserts that trading good and bad images of ethnically-labelled groups is 'essentialist': 'That is, positive images of black people assume that all black people have essential qualities in common. They may not' (Barker 1999: 218). Yet despite this empirical claim, he also writes: 'The strategy rests on an epistemology of realism by which it is thought possible to bring representations of black people into line with "real" black people. This is not viable, for the real is always already a representation.' This proposition, he implies, is consistent with his claim that '[r]epresentation is constitutive of race as cultural identity and not a mirror or distortion of it' (Barker 1999: 83).

This way of writing muddles semiotic and epistemological issues around race in the most confusing ways. Barker's analysis moves from 'black people' (whom he refers to as an actual group of humans) to race as 'cultural identity', which is reducible to 'representation'. It is not clear whether the mantra that 'the real is always already a representation' is meant to claim that real states of affairs, objects and processes, are in fact *all and only* 'representations', or whether a weaker claim is being made that is consistent with a less-obviously idealist epistemology.

Employing the concept of 'representation' must presuppose a medium and agent (presumably a human agent): representations do not float free of any material realization. How 'the real' could be coherently thought of as *only* ('always already') representation without postulating some omnipotent semiotician to represent it, so to speak, is hard to imagine. Moreover, one does not need to be too much of a literalist to ask how, in fact, 'representation' could 'constitute' ('cause' totally?) even the *cultural* identity of actual people. The infinite variety of individual subjectivities suggests that different narrativizations of social experiences are *causally* relevant to people's sense of who they are, but part of this process involves identifying with some but not other cultural groupings. This is not to deny that in specific cultural contexts skin colour or facial features *as represented* (and taken to mean) are an important factor both in how people understand 'race' and in determining some aspects of individual 'identity'.

Making Sense of Difference

I have considered social and semiotic constructionism at some length because it purports to displace all realist epistemologies, and because it cites putative race differences as examples of conceptual errors that need to be demystified through anti-realist analysis. The biggest error is 'essentialism' – the idea that classes of people share certain qualities and that these are immutable, part of their unchanging and unchangeable 'nature': differences are *caused by some hidden determinants* (hence race, sex or mental illness are postulated as causes without any evidential warrant). So 'naïve realists' assume that races are *real* – that there exist actual groups of different kinds of people, and that all the members of each group share particular attributes or qualities (their 'essence'). This notion is politically pernicious, because it leads to rac*ism* – the belief in essential (biological, unchangeable) differences between so-called races. Racism embodies the assumption that physical *differences* in variables such as skin colour, eye-shape etc. are not only real but indicate other, 'deeper' psychological or physical differences between *individuals*. This is a naïvely empiricist view, and it has been justifiably criticized by Cultural Studies writers, as it has by other social scientists, especially anthropologists, and by many biologists.

The push to avoid essentialism that led to the culturalist notion that race can be understood as a reaction to rigid essentialist and regressive politics of 1970s' psychobiology. The most controversial instance of this was the prominent British psychologist, Hans Eysenck's (1971) claim to have demonstrated racial differences in measurable 'intelligence'. In the seventies, even to debate the evidence adduced by Eysenck was seen to endorse his essentialist notion of race and hence, it was often claimed, his rac*ism*. However, the ontological status of the concept of race is not the *sine qua non* of whether it can be used for racist political purposes. 'Theory's' celebration of 'difference' as non-essentialist does not, *by itself*, guarantee liberal or progressive politics. It is not racist to allow that it is an *empirical question* whether one population of inter-breeding people exhibits different relative frequencies of some definable qualities when compared to another specified group.

Scientific comparisons of genetic differences define races in 'relative' ways: 'gene pools' or inter-breeding populations are studied comparatively and in numbers appropriate to observing the possible frequencies of the factors being observed. Unlike in Eysenck, this process is not post hoc. Scientific comparisons do *not assume* that *each member* of a specified interbreeding population exhibits any particuar characteristic, so they are not vulnerable to the criticism that they are essentialist or reductionist *as such*. And, of course, most, if not all, differences in the frequencies of observable factors between groups of people are of no scientific interest. Some, such as propensities to certain diseases or immunological defences, may be.

The lessons I hope to draw from my detailed analysis of the methodologocal/theoretical issues centred on the concept of 'race' and 'difference' are several. First, ethno-linguistic identity is not mapped onto biological features of groups of actual people in the way that everyday English implies. But that is not a matter that *by itself* undermines the value of biologically comparative and relative notions of race thought of as populations. Like those in the scientific (medical and anthropological) disciplines that also study human diversity and its causes, Cultural Studies Theorists of differen*ces* between various definable groups of people need to attend to the epistemological implications of their own theorizing: 'difference' is not a useful synonym for 'race', but *both* terms can be used meaningfully if each is clearly defined.

Second, it is important to note that rac*ism* is not *implied* by realist concepts of race any more than it is by relativist or social constructivist interpretations of the term. Acknowledging differences between groups of people has no implications for discriminating against or in favour of them, neither in social policy nor in everyday life. This can be seen by comparison with the example of a group of people whose obvious physical characteristics do *not* allow them to be classified as a group. What individual twins look like is totally irrelevant to their 'difference': identical twins, as a population, are reported to perform slightly but significantly below the average of singletons on psychological tests of 'intelligence' (Bell & Staines 2001: 181–88). However, this has no implications for how or whether twins should be treated differently from others in educational policy or legal rights. Acknowledging that differences are 'real' does not *imply* that any particular kind of discriminatory behaviour is justified.

Third, it is ironic that the laudable aim of analysing and describing all cultures without essentialist assumptions may have cost Cultural Studies the chance to argue more strongly against reductive biologism, against naïve empiricism – and therefore against racism. Race labelling is frequently conceptually confused, even illogical. Races are invoked to 'explain' post hoc (after the event, circularly or uninformatively) all and any aspects of individual and group behaviours. This usually amounts to no more than a rationalization for prejudice. Consider the two propositions, *Barak Obama intervened to support the US auto industry*; and *Barak Obama was a superb athlete at college*. To attribute either of these phenomena to Obama's 'race' is to offer only a *pseudo-explanation* of them. This is not because race is a social construct, but because *no causal factors* are implied in such accounts which invoke race in reductive and essentialist ways. If race is claimed to 'cause' particular behaviour, then, minimally, some race-correlated biological factors sufficient to bring about that behaviour would need to be postulated, and these should be observable independently of the behaviour they are said to cause (see Bell & Staines, 2001: 83–90 for a discussion of circular explanation in Psychology).

However, to claim that *all race concepts are social constructs* regardless of their contexts, and so to refuse to evaluate empirical claims about psychological, biological or cultural reality may be self-defeating and politically disempowering. Speaking about 'difference' in the abstract does not solve the conceptual problems that racism entails. It seems at best unhelpful always to relativize and subjectivize the putatively critical concept of race, for example, as do Wetherell and Potter (1992), as 'subjective … and continuously created intertextually'. Methodologically rigorous criticsm of racism (and sexism, for that matter) can be advanced without recourse to social/linguistic constructionism and to the epistemological relativism that this implies.

In this chapter I have tried to show that the care taken by Theorists to avoid an ontology of 'static phenomena', proposing instead the creative, fluid processes and 'becomings' favoured by Deleuze and recirculated by his enthusiastic Anglophone followers, may lead to a new kind of reification – that of 'difference' itself. Second, I have illustrated options for avoiding reductionist and essentialist practices in understanding cultural differences, recommending instead a realist foundation for critique. In both cases, I urge that participants involved in these difficult debates pay each other the courtesy of clearly and explicitly defining their terms.

Chapter 4

Theory, People and 'Subjects'

... we can rapidly change our bodies, cultures and subjectivities.
Andrew Murphie and John Potts

Psychology and the Emergence of Cultural Studies

The move towards a general semiotic description of clothing, cooking, myths and movies (to name but a few) is most celebrated in the early writings of the French *littérateur*, Roland Barthes. Semiotics (the general science of signs and their use) was shown by Barthes to yield genuine insights into an array of cultural phenomena. Others, such as Jacques Durand (1970), applied Ferdinand de Saussure's ideas to various cultural examples, such as modern display advertising, showing that they constituted a system or a structured set of interrelated elements.

By the 1980s, Anglophone literary, semiotic and cultural studies had discovered the new, more abstract, even metaphysical implications of the French Theorists, Derrida, and later, Deleuze. Meanwhile, the English linguist, Michael Halliday, theorized all speech as socially contextualized *action*. Soon visual and musical 'texts' (popular and high art), as well as literary works, had been ground through the structuralist, and then the post-structuralist, mills of academe. The result was a heady brew indeed, especially for an undergraduate in Melbourne, Minnesota or Manchester, who probably thought 'structuralism' was a branch of engineering.

Anglo-American Psychology was also under attack – from Marxism, Feminism, and 'anti-psychiatry' movements – to name only the most obvious. The post-war expansion of university education had seen huge numbers of hapless humanities students respectably schooled in Psychology, albeit an innocently empirical, eclectically humanistic psychology. The new critics saw in this 'science', conformism and intellectual timidity, positivism and political conservatism. So not only the French 'Left' flirted with existentialist psychology, Lacanian psychoanalysis, or sought to analyse the politics of 'identity' in terms of communication and language. At more or less the same time, in the United States and in Britain, conventional psychiatry and psychology, aimed at 'adjusting' people to 'reality', were increasingly derided. Thomas Szasz, RD Laing, Gregory Bateson, and others agreed with the French critics of psychiatric models of 'normality' and opposed the psychiatrically-sanctioned control of 'patients'. Mental illness was a 'myth', said Szasz; 'asylums' were merely prisons reinforcing the deadening conformity of other institutions like the school and family. Some strands of Psychology moved away from biological, causal and normative models, part of the accelerating antagonism to 'empiricism' (usually labelled 'positivism') in European social theory.

'Radical' psychologists and anti-psychiatrists worked in the margins of biologically-oriented and behaviouristic 'schools'. They attracted many followers during the 1960s and 1970s who came to regard Psychology as at best trivial, at worst politically repressive. To the extent that Cultural Studies addressed explicitly psychological questions, it also did so from these radically critical standpoints. It gravitated towards humanities rather than social or biological science traditions, preferring phenomenological and hermeneutic concepts for describing the nuances of cultural experience. Emerging Feminisms also rejected biological 'essentialism'; literature courses celebrated readers' diverse uses of texts, and re-analysed the ideological import of the literary 'canon': because interpretation presupposed one valid meaning for a text, it was argued, it could all too easily become hegemonic, denying minority and subaltern experience.

Within this foment, ethnic, linguistic, and gendered 'identities' and 'difference' (in the abstract, meaning 'diversity' of identity) were *celebrated* rather than *explained*. Experience, not meaning; difference not essence; verbs, not nouns; affects and effects, not motives and causes – these preferences came to drive Cultural Studies discourse by the end of the twentieth century. Although it adopted 'Theory' based on revised psychoanalysis and metaphysics, Cultural Studies branched off from the Anglo-American disciplines of psychology, sociology and anthropology to constitute a distinct field of interdisciplinary study. Here its methodologies became self-consciously 'semiotic' and its ambition hardened into critique of established disciplines and of their epistemological complacency. In these ways it continued the de- and re-construction of the humanities and social sciences begun on the Left Bank and Berkeley in the 1960s. Amongst the paradigm shifts and political movements were: 'Deconstruction' (à la Derrida); Semio-psychoanalysis (à la Lacan); Post-Colonialism (France 'lost' its colonies during the 1950s); various Feminisms; Marxist sociological exposés of capitalist 'hegemony'; and US antiwar and counter-culture Libertarianism. These formed the context – the pre-history – of what would be called Cultural Studies from the 1980s.

The 'Return to the Signifier'

'Semiotics' is the general name given to those theories that analyse signs and codes and seek to understand how meaning is transacted in social life. Linguistics is a branch of Semiotics. So too are systems of analysis aimed at showing how *visual* 'texts' allow people in a cultural context to share and dispute meanings amongst themselves. Semiotics is concerned with how texts (whether linguistic or not) can be said to 'work'. As all meaning is sociocultural, semiotics has become a central component of Cultural Studies.

The relationships amongst Semiotics and more established hermeneutic and social science disciplines remain ill-defined and are frequently antagonistic. This is despite works such as Umberto Eco's (2000) excursion into analytical philosophy and various forays into psychoanalysis (following Lacan) as well as recent re-theorizations of questions once the sole province of empirical psychology (such as questions of individual identity or even language development). In the Anglophone academies at least, the older disciplines continue to theorize and apply their various knowledges more or less unperturbed by the suspicion that all these activities are just discursive rehearsals of their own unreflective ignorance. They do not anxiously await enlightenment from the sons and daughters of Saussure. The 'semiotic turn' in the humanities has not really altered the epistemological or ontological assumptions of existing disciplines so much as opened up new inter- or cross-disciplinary specializations which sometimes sit rather uneasily beside their older siblings, often failing to communicate with them in productive ways.

My interest in semiotic theorizations of subjectivity is limited to their specifically psychological and epistemological implications. This chapter considers typical Cultural Studies claims in which aspects of psychological phenomena like perception, emotional responses, personal identity or subjectivity (in general) are putatively explained *by* semiological phenomena, or explained *as* semiological phenomena. Although such accounts are not necessarily reductionist or circular, in many historically important examples they can be seen to be inadequate and question-begging. Semiological and culturalist accounts make claims that are contrary to (and may sometimes contradict) the kinds of empirical accounts of many phenomena found in disciplines like Psychology or Anthropology. Leaving aside the adequacy of the latter approaches, I caution against too-ready and uncritical acceptance of semiotic accounts (by which I mean, ultimately, explanatory analyses, including empirical descriptions) of psychological phenomena. I will discuss several examples of recent semiological and of post-structuralist accounts of what I think it is reasonable to label 'psychological' phenomena, in that they involve human cognition, learning or adaptation to the social or physical environment, and/or because they postulate notions of human 'agency'.

Semiotic Subjects, or Persons?

> In the introduction to *The Psychic Life of Power* Judith Butler concludes: '… we must lose the perspective of a subject already formed in order to account for our own becoming. That 'becoming' is no simple or continuous affair, but an uneasy practice of repetition and its risks, compelled yet incomplete, wavering on the horizon of social being'. In a later study Colebrook suggests that we can conceive of 'becoming as an actualization and enchantment or enrichment of being' (Colebrook, 2002, p. 90) … The presenters in this symposium will draw on a range of theorists in order to further explicate the idea of 'becoming' and consider how it might be employed to enrich our efforts teaching and writing in the fields of Cultural Studies and Education. (Cultural Studies Association, 2003: 15)

This rather typical example of Cultural Studies discourse refers to the 'subject', suggests how it is formed (it speaks of accounts of people's actual 'becoming') and then promises discussion of the value of this concept in Education and in Cultural Studies. Yet Cultural Studies is rather ambivalent about the value of, indeed the possibility of, studying what at school we used to call 'human beings'.

> We need first to understand that the human form – including human desire and all its external representations – may be changing rapidly, and thus must be re-visioned. We need to understand that five hundred years of humanism may be coming to an end as humanism transforms itself into something that we must helplessly call post-humanism. (Ihab Hassan, quoted in Hayles 1999b: 1)

Both of these unexceptional quotes from the Cultural Studies literature of the past decade refer to *psychological* phenomena, pointing to variables that need to be considered in explanatory accounts of human psychological change. The descriptions of desiring, 'becoming' (changing?) beings so beloved of recent Cultural Studies are ironically reminiscent of what used to be called 'humanistic psychology'. Readers trained in academic psychology who read the above might be reminded that, in the 1960s particularly, 'humanistic' psychologists opposed all manner of deterministic, behaviouristic, Freudian and biologistic approaches to studying and counselling real people. People, they asserted, should be seen neither as machines nor as animals; they were uniquely 'human'. Writers such as Abraham Maslow and Carl Rogers spoke of a drive towards 'self-actualization' that they saw as an innate propensity in people, a motive that could explain psychological growth and openness to new, liberating experience. The anxieties attendant on the hierarchy of social and biological drives could be overcome, or so Rogerian therapy assured the clients on whom it was centred. Essentially, the 'client' was counselled to 'know her or his-self'.

As discussed in Chapters 1 and 2, the concept of 'becoming' may have been a metaphysical concept in its original Deleuzian context. However, when it found its way into English academic discourse, it has often been translated into a prosaic psychological register. This psychological (and, I would say, deterministic) sense is implied in the above quotation from the Cultural Studies Conference abstract. It trades on the ambiguity of the term, and psychologizes it to explain the process of 'becoming subjects'. But this seems a trivial use: it hardly helps to understand 'how individuals develop subjectivities and sexual and gender identities' (Rasmussen abstract CSA 2003: 15). That is, 'becoming' seems merely to refer to psychological development or to changes culminating in a preferred (enriched) being or identity. Self-actualization, perhaps, despite the new vocabulary.

A significant strand of orthodox Cultural Studies Theory explicitly challenges empirical Psychology. If psychology is defined as the *study of the nature and causes of (human) behaviour in its social contexts*, then biosocial determinism, including explanations formulated in terms of motivation, for example, will be central to its discourse. Psychology postulates a more or less coherent human 'subject' or identity, centred on memory and agency. The discipline assumes that 'people' can be described in terms of actual, unique identities, and as 'objects' with certain qualities or characteristics, both as species and as individuals. And, because all people are necessarily social entities, they inhabit and express 'culture' (the symbolic meanings and values of the various social aggregations with which they 'identify').

Culturally-embedded psychological identities are therefore the object that is taken for granted in what became, during the late nineteenth and twentieth centuries, the discipline of empirical Psychology. As does folk psychology, post-Enlightenment academic psychology accepts a naturalistic, not a supernatural or religious concept of the person, and assumes that people's behavioural particularities can, in principle, be rationally, and that means deterministically, explained (within practical limits). A necessary aspect of such explanation is causation. A necessary object of study is the human nervous system (including the brain, of course).

It comes as a surprise to read, under the banner of Cultural Studies, 'Theoretical' writing that rejects all or most of these assumptions and celebrates novel ways of understanding the nature and causes of psychological identity. Theory is often explicitly anti-humanistic and proudly antagonistic to the 'anthropocentrism' of conventional psychology (see Chapter 5). This position is as odd as a religious approach to psychology that postulates 'souls', 'free will' and morality as its focus. It certainly surprises most students who innocently assume that *human* psychology is by definition anthropocentric. Nevertheless, many recent Theorists, citing 'post-structuralism' as their guide, propose that human agency is little more than a linguistic convenience. Some claim that non-human and even inorganic matter (!) can be analysed in the same metaphorical ways as animal and human 'life'.

Cultural Studies is frequently written on the assumption that Psychology's claim to being 'scientific' is fraudulent, and that subjects, not people, must be postulated to allow their culturally determined 'identities' to be conceptualized and understood. And 'the subject' in general, is created in and through 'discourse', it is asserted. Theory's claims amount to a semiologically inspired and thus culturally deterministic attempt to change the concept of the subject within realist psychology. Theory argues that psychology is *reducible* to 'meaning', in that the subject of what was once psychology is actually, so to speak, a position or point (a 'subject position') in a network of ever-changing signs systems. This move is what some commentators, most notably Terry Eagleton (1997), have called 'culturalism' (the reduction of all psychological and political matters to cultural and linguistic/semiotic phenomena). Like me, most students are interested in actual people, and in what causes them to be the way they are. The extent to which people's identities or subjectivities are formed by their cultural experiences and semiotic 'ecologies', they might agree, is an empirical question – a question of evidence. Both biology and acculturation give rise to semiotic subjectivity.

Decentring Psychology

The principal argument advanced in Cultural Studies' accounts of subjectivity and identity amount to the following: if cultures consist of 'texts', 'signs' and 'discourse', and people are defined as cultural entities, then semiotic concepts can be proposed as necessary and (perhaps) sufficient for such traditionally psychologically-defined phenomena as individual 'identity' and gender. As this is central to Theory that underpins much of Cultural Studies, and as it figures in undergraduate textbooks, I will consider the question of how (or *whether*) semiotic theories provide necessary or sufficient analysis of 'subjectivity' in general – that is, of what it means to 'be a subject'. It will help the reader if I indicate that the term 'subject' is used in many ways, and that in some writing it is still simply equated with the 'person' or the 'agent' or the 'ego'. That is, it is merely a new name for the psychological individual.

'Subjectivity' can mean 'the subjective realm' – the realm of all the perception events and semiotic events (including utterances) to which the personal pronouns 'I' and/or 'we' could be applied. So reports of one's dreams, one's engagement with a film or piece of music, one's decoding a sentence, etc. are all 'subjective'. And, on some accounts, these events (and nothing more) *constitute* 'the subject'. Following Lacan (and Althusser) Cultural Theorists have proposed that 'the subject' is no more than a 'semiotic position', the 'I-centre' where the body-image mirrored back from 'outside' (from the mirror of the social other) gives linguistic agency to the subject. The subject is 'called up', 'called into existence through', or addressed as already part of, semiosis. Referring to Foucault, Horst Ruthrof has written:

> Foucault draws our attention away from the subject as psychologically complex entity and towards questions such as Who is speaking? Who is qualified to speak? Who receives prestige from speaking? Who is sanctioned by law or tradition to speak? From what site is she or he speaking? From within which kind of institution? (Ruthrof 2000: 197–8)

So, following this line, the decentred, non-psychological (certainly non-biological) concept has been abstracted to the point where 'subject positions' are postulated. These are said to be constructed through semiosis (and they are usually rather vaguely specified as 'discursive'). For example, gendered 'subject positions' (sometimes simply called 'gendered subjects') are claimed to be sociological/discursive, and not psychobiological. They are defined relationally, not essentially. However, as will become clear later, the concept cannot adequately be defined in this way. To anticipate the problems I see, consider Guatarri's oddly circular definition. He characterizes subjectivity (in general, so to speak) as follows:

> The ensemble of conditions which render possible the emergence of individual and/ or collective instances of self-referential existential territories, adjacent or in a delimiting relation to an alterity that is itself subjective. (Guatarri 1995: 9)

If we are to take Guattari at his word, he wants 'subjectivity' to refer not to any entity and/ or to its qualities and the relationships that obtain between it and other entities or processes but to relations and conditions themselves, even though these seem to have no empirical reference or import. Even on a more generous interpretation, he seems to define subjectivity in several ways: as either individual or collective and inter-subjectively, yet from the 'outside'. Like Lacan and Foucault, he emphasizes 'alterity', although in an apparently different role. And as with Lacan, the pronominal or self-referential aspect of the 'subject in general' or what might be called 'subject-hood' or 'subject-ness' is emphasized. The child identifies its image in the mirror, but before it can use language this apparent object is a thing like any other and is named accordingly as an 'object'. But the child is subjected to, and becomes the first person pronominal subject of, language thereby becoming 'a subject'. It is both object and subject, and by using language substitutes 'I' or 'me' for its proper name. Before this development, children use their own name in the third person: 'Lara want to play', 'Johnny hate apples'.

So the subjective realm (including that of humans' experiences/perceptions or sensations) has been radically re-theorized in semiotic terms to the point where individual psychological subjects are principally understood as pronouns that operate at discursive intersections, to put the matter crudely. Such a theory analyses what it might be better to call '*subject-hood*' (that is, it postulates the conditions for being a 'subject in general') via processes of subjectivation through language. However, Cultural Studies writers frequently equivocate by using the term 'subject' as synonymous with actual *persons*, i.e. as 'subjects' in the commonsense meaning of the term. Hence Judith Butler is quoted (above) referring to 'our own becoming' thereby assuming a psychobiological entity which is changing (which is subject to change, so to speak).

Equivocating: Anti-'Essentialism'

What I call equivocation about the concept of the subject is most blatant in Cultural Studies textbooks. Consider briefly the theoretical and empirical adequacy of two typical summary accounts of the 'social production' of what is termed either 'subjectivity' or 'identity' – first from Barker, *Television, Globalisation and Cultural Identities* (1999), and second from Schirato and Yell, *Communication and Cultural Literacy: An Introduction* (2000).

With the apparent aim of avoiding 'essentialism' when addressing the question 'what is a woman?' [*sic*] Barker (1999: 86) proposes that '… identities based on sex and gender are socially produced descriptions with which we identify and not universal categories of nature or metaphysics', and that one relevant factor in the circulation of such 'descriptions' is television culture: 'The representations of gender which television produces and circulates are themselves constitutive of gender as a cultural identity.' Note that Barker gives a crude causal account of 'identity' that involves people identifying with 'descriptions', although why one person would identify with one set of descriptions and not others, is not stated. Presumably that would either require a psychological hypothesis or it would involve the circular notion that the identity-defining needs of some identities cause them to identify with certain rewarding descriptions found in their particular culture but not with others Yet, like Butler above, Barker tries to avoid postulating actual persons who 'have' such identities. Instead 'representation' as such constitutes aspects of identity. Hence, the identities are themselves only circulating 'descriptions'. One might ask who or what are the 'we' involved in this bloodless process?

Barker seems to want to avoid any deterministic implications altogether, so he equates 'identity' with what he labels 'subjectivity'. He wants this move to allow him to smuggle in what he calls (human) agency. And he needs such agency to avoid the implications of the 'socially produced descriptions' (above) actually *determining*, in a circular way, whether or not we 'identify' with them. He fails to ask why 'we' (presumably already constituted or identifying and identified 'subjects') should *choose* (or be forced by circumstance to 'choose') one gendered description over all the others circulating in the culture. Hence this account begs the question of just how identity is formed in actual persons.

To try to move out of this circle, Barker invokes a rather indeterministic, even contradictory notion: he comments, '[o]ver all, what is being argued for … is the, in principle, infinite plasticity of human sexuality and gender…' (1999: 91).

In this account, the failure to distinguish sufficient conditions (causal factors) from necessary conditions, each related to precisely defined effects, leads to further confusions about subjectivity and/or identity. So Barker is forced to introduce a more agent-like term. He states: 'Indeed, the very idea of an intentional, sexed actor is a discursive production of performativity itself' (1999: 94). But by this point the conceptual field has become very muddy indeed. Now the cause and the effect, as well as the analytical distinctions they depend on, collapse into what is likely to be a nightmare for the undergraduate reader. Barker also quotes Butler: '… thus, gender is performative in the sense that it constitutes *as an effect* that very subject it appears to express' (1999: 24). It is not clear whether Barker believes that 'gender' *constitutes* or otherwise causes 'gendered subjects', but then it is unclear how to interpret the empirical import of such an apparently circular and vague claim. Of course, Butler adds a psychoanalytic dimension to her analysis but this centres on 'identification' anyway so we are back with Barker's initial problem.

While Barker effectively begs the question concerning the contingent empirical relationships that could hold between discourse and subjectivity, or 'descriptions/ representations' and identities, Schirato and Yell (2000) hint at a psychologically relevant, motivational feature of the processes discussed above. They offer 'desire' as the driver of action within the semiologially determined (or at least partially constituted) subject. Schirato and Yell argue that culture, such as popular magazines (they discuss *Dolly*), provides what might be called scripts through which people rehearse/perform their 'subjectivities' (and, like Barker, they also invoke Butler). But they allow both the 'misperformance' and the 'over-performance' of such culturally significant roles as 'femininity' and 'masculinity' (Schirato & Yell 2000: 101). So it is difficult to decide whether such performances are merely *necessary* or are *sufficient* for the constitution of gendered identity. This is because to claim that someone can *over*perform an identity presumes that it is definable normatively and that it is not itself causal of the person's behaviour. To put this crudely, what entity or what identity could be postulated as doing the over- or the mis-performing of identity-defining scripts (Barker's 'descriptions')?

According to Schirato and Yell: '… people don't just conform to the ideas and imperatives coming out of the media, advertising and government'. They allow that it is 'people' who perform, and thus, they cannot, by definition, be synonymous with 'subjectivities' as such. Yet Schirato and Yell also claim that 'subjects' are 'able to pick and choose, and incorporate different aspects of subjectivity in order to commoditize themselves' (2000: 105). So in their analysis, 'people' *are and are not* equated with 'subjects' and the latter are sometimes at least seen as capable of agency (of 'acting … in order to …'). The authors go on to say that subjects are always '… split because they are partly constituted out of repressed or unconscious desire', although that only seems to compound their difficulties (2000: 105).

Clearly, Shirato and Yell echo Judith Butler's analyses of gendered identity, although they also dilute it somewhat. In her discussion of 'identity, sex and the metaphysics of substance', Butler asks:

> What can be meant by 'identity', then, and what grounds the presumption that identities are self-identical [sic], persisting through time as the same, unified and internally coherent?

She then argues that the discussion of identity

> ought not to proceed prior to a discussion of gender identity for the simple reason that 'persons' only become intelligible through becoming gendered in conformity with recognisable standards of gender intelligibility. (1990: 16)

She points out that agency and stability understood as residing 'inside' the organism have been conventionally agreed as the defining characteristics of a 'person', but she objects that this ignores the extent to which 'identity' is a 'normative ideal, rather than a descriptive feature of experience' (1990: 16). She warns against a fixed, stipulative empirical definition of gender and hence of identity (against the 'normative telos of definitional closure' to use her words).

Insofar as Butler allows that identity and persons are, so to speak, negotiated between the biological entity and its discursive or social environment, one can have no quibbles with her general position. Further, the identities in question do not remain the fixed causes of their own expression, but are continuously expressed or 'realized' (my term, not hers) through social engagement or negotiation. She seeks to avoid attributing fixed, 'essentialist' qualities to gendered identity, to avoid describing an object, because this would essentialize and reify (or 'thingify') the concept. Nevertheless, a psychologist might judge that this subtlety downplays the actual *causal* factors that could be relevant to how identity is developed and expressed in individual cases.

The laudable emphasis on 'becoming' and 'change' may have been bought at the cost of any reference to specific causal factors, such as an individual's actual history of physical pleasurable or painful experiences and their social meanings (as Freud would have emphasized, for instance). The 'body' that permeates the semiotic/cultural and relativistic discussions of gendered identity and personhood following Butler (who was heavily influenced by Foucault) seems hardly to be recognizably material, let alone visceral and dynamic. The events of their respective histories seem not to be remembered in terms of the drives or motives of the various bodies. Yet this is exactly what a psychological understanding of identity would usually attend to. Psychological accounts of personal identity – gendered, aged, 'raced' – all need to take into account the discursive or cultural factors that theorists such as Butler emphasize. However, 'identities' are not, therefore, *completely reducible* to semiotic or cultural determination, even allowing for the fact that cultural norms and descriptions must be considered when they are described.

Although Cultural Studies draws attention to aspects of the material and semiotic contexts in which identities 'grow' or develop, and tries to avoid essentialism, this does not render its accounts immune to empirical evaluation – to evidence. To take an illuminating example: 'schizophrenic' identities were, until quite recently, thought to result entirely from 'disorders of communication'. Schizophrenic 'subjectivity' expressed ways by which people coped with extremely disorienting communication, such as habitual contradictory injunctions from family members. We might have said that experiences and behaviours labelled schizophrenic were constructed through discourse, quite literally. But this has proven to be wrong. Evidence of neurobiological causal factors has been discovered. This makes a great difference to the sense of what it means to be, or to be a family member of, a 'schizophrenic' person.

What I have called 'culturalism' and 'semiotic determinism' must be seen as *hypotheses* about what causal factors are contingently relevant to the actual differences between people, their subjectivities and identities. Psychology is concerned with both subjective aspects (what it is feels like to 'be' a person, whatever label society attaches to this) and with identity considered objectively as knowable aspects of a person's behavioural predispositions, temperament, values, etc. Equivocal and vague 'culturalist' analyses, to put my position most strongly, seem to have arisen to cover the lack of an adequate, causal account of subjectivity and of particular aspects (such as gendered aspects) of identity or identities (by which I mean individual people's identities). Seeing 'subjects' as some kind of *tabula rasa* onto which the culture writes its meanings is both too simplistically 'strong' (it predicts a passive, narrow range of clones) and is, in its own way, 'reductionist', with subjective qualities now reducible to the body's culture rather than being explained by the person's particular biology and biography.

Subjects Need Biology

It is not my aim here to provide alternative analyses of identity or subjectivity. It should be clear from the above that this would mean presenting various focused, psychological theories supported by evidence. Instead, I have restricted my critique to some recent approaches that have most obviously reduced what I see as psychological, causal accounts of psychological identity to vaguely semiotic interpretations. Of course, my cautionary points do not imply that the cited theorists are *generally* misguided. That would be a stronger claim and require different argument.

To suggest what kinds of concepts would be necessary for an adequate explanatory account of such psychological complexities, let me at least briefly indicate some alternative but, I believe, necessary assumptions. Ironically these are from a (once-was) Marxist literary theorist, Terry Eagleton. Eagleton defends a modified 'essentialism', and cuts through semiotic reductionism (although he does not call it by that name) by arguing that humans are *more than sign-determined* (a view that he terms 'culturalism'). 'Culturalism is quite as much a form of reductionism as biologism', he asserts (Eagleton 1997: 74), arguing that humans must be thought of as having a 'nature'. This founding assumption is consistent with Hirsch, who concludes his study of physical and psychological identity by also criticising semiotic, conventionalist accounts:

> The alternative to conventionalism … consists in the following hypothesis: We conceive of the self as we do because this is a kind of psychological necessity … it is basic to human nature … It is a more or less specialized and irreducible fact about our nature that we think of the self as we do. (Hirsch 1982: 302)

By contrast to the Cultural Studies accounts of subjects, which seem to describe at best an anodyne, idealist phenomenon, many theorists writing within Psychology and Analytical Philosophy accept that biological factors interact with particular semiotic and other experiential factors to 'make' identities what they are. Griffiths (1997) proposes as essential to understanding human psychology a realist concept of 'emotions'. Freud could be said to offer a realist approach as well: he postulated a biological substrate that is differentiated into culturally distinct patterns of temperament and emotion through an individual's experiences. Further, he proposed dynamic, causal processes, such as 'identification' with others as what partly determines personality differences. Unlike Butler, however, Freudian theory emphasized the 'ego-defensive' functions of identification and the rewards and anxieties in which it is enmeshed in particular people's lives. Historically, psychologists have seen the 'ego' as a complex and determining system rather than as a screen onto which cultural signs are projected, and have analysed individual dispositions to behave and 'personalities' (now a quaintly archaic term) as a function of motives, needs, learned modes of response (conditioned by pleasure/pain). To say identity is 'embodied' (as does Theory) ought surely to attend to how the body remembers and interprets its motivated interactions with culture.

Psychologists have to confront the impossibility of explaining identit*ies* by deploying the one conveniently general concept of ident*ity*. They have not clutched at glib or circular notions such as 'difference' or 'subjectivity' as convenient simplifications of causal factors involved in psychological explanation. Just as much as Cultural Studies commentators, many psychologists see subjective conflict, unconscious identifications, etc., as part of the dynamic explanation of identity. Messy concepts like drives and habits, memory and emotions, needs and attitudes, are needed if we are to understand why actual people are as they are, and, indeed why human cultures take the forms they do:

> '… we are not 'cultural' rather than 'natural' creatures, but cultural creatures by virtue of our natures, which is to say by virtue of the sorts of bodies we have and the kinds of world to which they belong. (Eagleton 1996: 72–73)

Psychological *identities*, by definition, persist through time, although continuously changing and, perhaps, settling into periodic 'stages'. Identities have a kind of 'career' (to quote Hirsch) as discrete and continuing entities. Psychological entities adapt to circumstances, learn and remember; they interact with, and are changed by, environmental/cultural/technological contingencies.

Not surprisingly, then, psychologists have proposed many differing kinds of explanations for such (id)entities and for their defining behavioural differences. Bell and Staines (2001) discuss the principal classes of psychological explanation, cautioning against circular and reductionist 'explanations'. They list 'folk-narrative', genetic (evolutionary), functional, teleological, componential, dispositional, connectionist, and other types of explanation for various psychological phenomena. It is ironic that the kinds of semiotic reductionism that I have criticized in this chapter arose as critiques of psychological determinism and essentialism (particularly biological essentialism). The critics have failed to appreciate the complexities of psychological phenomena and undervalued empirically-circumscribed analysis and explanation based on detailed descriptions of the explananda (the phenomena to be explained) and the explanans (the putatively explanatory proposals). Yet these are the very stuff of modern psychology.

As an alternative to psychological theory, semiotic culturalism may offer only reductive, simplistic explanatory potential, and may even prove quite vacuous or circular in many contexts. Despite its enthusiasm for the kinds of idealist psychological concepts I have discussed in this chapter, recent Cultural Studies offers no good arguments for throwing out the idea that each flesh-and-blood person is a particular, actual psychological entity. Yes, we need to conceive of them as subjects (language users, 'I-centres' or 'I-dentities') but also as people who are conflict-prone, complexly motivated, pleasure-seeking and pain-avoiding *animals*. Replacing this way of describing psychosocial entities by abstract semiotic terminologies solves no metaphysical problems. To describe persons as semiotic subjects and nothing more is not only what Theorists themselves call reductive, it begs the question of what *caused* them to be *who and what* they individually become.

As a post-script to this discussion, I draw Cultural Studies readers to books such as *Altered Egos: How the Brain Creates the Self* by Todd Feinberg (2001) that provide non-semiological, but quite subtle accounts of how individual organisms cohere as 'identities'. Feinberg even addresses Cartesian dualism and the question of how subjectivity coheres around an 'I' or ego. I am surprised that academics interested in educating their students about culture, meaning, subjectivity and identity feel the need to invoke 'self-referential existential territories' and the like when more prosaic but coherent accounts of these issues are available in English anyway. Moreover, sociology, literature, media and culture students seem to have coped with their disciplines for decades without having to adhere to any particular metaphysical solution to these problems. Certainly, they have felt no need to reinvent Psychology and Neurology to pursue their various academic interests in the humanities and social sciences.

My critic might reply that Theory of subjectivity and identity is not intended to complete with the accounts offered in Psychology or Neuroscience. Biology has nothing to do with the issues discussed in this chapter, if one accepts this argument. But to do so would surely be quite disingenuous. The examples discussed here and in other chapters are put forward by their respective authors as ways of criticizing and improving on psychological theory and its philosophical assumptions (foundations). Unless Theorists explicitly opt out of academic debate by claiming to write figuratively or imaginatively without the need to refer to knowable features of reality, they must countenance rational counter-argument. Their students should expect nothing less.

Chapter 5

'Post-Human' Theory and Cultural Studies

Nature, Mr. Allnut, is what we are put into the world to rise above.
                                    'The African Queen' (John Huston) 1951

Man is something to be overcome.
                                    Nietzsche

The Printing Press, Digital Media and Humanism

The telescope and the *camera obscura*, the daguerreotype and the movie camera provided models and metaphors for vision and memory during the Industrial Age. Today, digital information-processing and storage devices (computers), their intimate psychological implications and their global social uses, furnish richly-suggestive metaphors and models for psychobiological speculation and have fuelled the literary and cinematic imagination. Cultural Studies emerged as a response not only to the disciplines that it criticized and sought to transcend but also as a series of conversations about revolutionary developments in digital technologies. These involve innovative aesthetic, psychological and communicational models and invite biological speculation. Long-accepted philosophical concepts have been revised and rethought. Perhaps the most radical of these re-imaginings for media and Cultural Studies have been the concept of the 'post-human' and its bastard siblings. What these problematic concepts might actually refer to, and how they have been used in argument against the humanities disciplines and their methodological assumptions, are questions central to the post-disciplinary academy. They threaten the very bases of humanistic scholarship undermining post-Enlightenment epistemological, ethical and ontological certainties. 'Virtual realities', virtual bodies, prosthetic information devices, 'second lives', etc. at least *sound* as though they promise or threaten new kinds of experiences and even new kinds of beings. Digitization foretells a brave new world-view in which humans will no longer be at the centre of what is knowable or valuable.

In *Orality and Literacy* Walter Ong has written with great insight about the development of humanistic (including, ultimately, secular) individualism. Insisting that media are not reducible to inventions of discrete physical technologies, he argues that media emerge from the convergence of technologies within evolving cultural/political institutions – the printing press merged movable type with the purposes and cultures of the church, initially at least, helping to construct privatistic, individualistic and, ultimately, secular, subjects. Five hundred years later the computer (itself made up in part of a typewriter and a video screen) is a portal to the libraries of the world, to all the information (if not knowledge) that can be inter-subjectively communicated.

A vulgar version of these ideas was popularized by Marshall McLuhan, throughout the sixties especially. His mantra that the medium was the message provoked attention to the ways by which the media extend our bodies and minds, rather than merely provide information and experiences. The media make us different people as we are socially and cognitively 'extended'. Unlike McLuhan, Ong tried to provide precise evidence for the psychological and cultural consequences of literacy. Of course, literacy is implicated in all socio-historical change since the Renaissance, so the printing press is not to be thought of as a medium *directly* changing subjectivity/psychology.

The computer provides people with what are often called 'affordances' – ways of thinking and creating, of playing and communicating – that are genuinely irreducible to those of its component parts. It offers fascinated and compulsive engagement in gleaming idealizations of the carnal and the consumable, of the forgettable and the useful. It is not quite like any earlier technology, yet it is in some senses a communications medium. Perhaps its main feature is its curiously intangible renditions of the cultural plenitude of what seems like the whole of the world. If media are 'extensions of man' (*pace* McLuhan), then the new computer-mediated world is virtually [sic] infinite and our subjectivities are limited only by the finite time of our ever-decaying bodies.

Ong emphasized that print was temporally insistent, informationally precise, interiorized, and abstract. It made words into 'things'. Print helped describe the truth of the world. By contrast, digital network media seem to distribute subjectivity beyond the body; they are spatially and temporally unbounded, inter-subjective, rather than individualistic. All virtual worlds are commensurate with one another; truth seems irrelevant as they encode and network information as *experience*, rather than as reference to a non-semiotized 'real' world.

Enlightenment Human*ism*

Humanist values and ethical principles depend on a universalistic (or at least generalized) notion of the species called 'human'. Post-humanist Cultural Studies writers argue that universalism is an idealist myth and, therefore, that ethical or political humanism will be transcended as histories and cultures change. Indeed, a revolutionary expansion of ideas about 'what humans are' is being radically accelerated by new technological developments. Universalism and its attendant anthropocentric world-views are contingent on socio-cultural and technological contexts, it is assumed. In this, the post-humanists follow Marx and reject Rousseau. Indeed, even Darwin and Freud are dismissed for believing in essentialist notions of 'the human' or 'human nature'. Diversity and change, 'difference' and 'becoming' seem to displace these older, fixed and deterministic assumptions. So humanism is linked to actual techno-cultural conditions, and seen as an historically-grounded ideology or world-view. Thus, it is a contingent episteme or paradigm, and will fade away as its supporting conditions change.

However, the link between humanism and ideas about the nature of humans or their successors is far from clear in the Cultural Studies literature. Post-human*ism* is not necessarily focused on empirical claims about post-humanity:

> We need first to understand that the human form – including human desire and all its external representations – may be changing rapidly, and thus must be re-visioned. We need to understand that five hundred years of humanism may be coming to an end as humanism transforms itself into something that we must helplessly call post-humanism. (Ihab Hassan in Hayles 1999: 1)

What Hassan finds problematic in post-Renaissance Western culture, science and philosophy, here labelled 'humanism', is, of course, the epistemological focus on people as agents, as subjects of knowledge and as objects of the same. Theodore Schatzki (2002) calls this 'residual humanism'. Humanism in this sense displaces Christian world-views. Instead of a deity orchestrating the music of the spheres, the mundane naked ape struggles to create music in a finite material world. Post-humanism seems to wish this un-heroic species away. As I shall describe, influential Cultural Studies writers predict the demise of the assumed individualistic subject-as-knower, and the displacement of individual psychological agency generally (for reasons also discussed in Chapter 3). 'Human desire and all its external representations' (people's motives and their cultures?) that ground the Enlightenment view of humanism are as relativistic and socially determined as were their religious predecessors or equivalents in the days of alchemy and witchcraft, it is argued.

The relationships between humans and humanisms are complex and murky. So I will try to unravel some of these in the following. I will try to show that cultural commentators who speak as though 'persons' are excess conceptual baggage, that what we think of as 'people', 'persons', 'humans' and 'human subjects' are conceptually optional because human cultures are changing rapidly, are at best conceptually muddled.

Theodore Schatzki defends what he calls a 'residual humanism' in which human agency is central (2002: 193). He summarizes several sociological theorizations: for example, 'Value Humanism' is 'the thesis that humans, as opposed to God, being the order of the cosmos, or the structure of reason, are responsible for political-ethical values.' Yet he argues that humans are not 'the masters of both their psyches and the phenomena of meaning and intentionality'. This he calls 'Psychological Humanism', but he warns: '[T]he human mind cannot be considered the exclusive place of knowledge.' Schatzki rejects as well, because it is essentialist, what he calls 'Definitional Humanism' – 'the thesis that human life essentially contrasts with or differs absolutely from animality or animal life.'

We can see here that all brands of humanisms attribute various real qualities to humans as a species. In common parlance, of course 'Humanism' refers to a range of overlapping views centred on the belief that human beings have value in themselves, and are not part of any divine plan. This is the source of all civic values and rights. Second, science and reason are assumed to be capable of providing comprehensive explanations of the universe and human life itself. So, humanism(s) reject(s) myth and religion as epistemologies and ontologies (Bullock & Trombley 2000: 406).

Humanists generally would claim that their position rests on much more than the belief that humans are simply a unique species. But it does assume this, so recent Theorists of the 'post-human' frequently extend their views to claim that that all Humanisms are passé because the species cannot be defined in the ways that secular scientific rationalists have assumed. Not only is the human species not unique in any metaphysical or religious sense, it is itself continuously changing into a new set of technologically-augmented beings (becoming post-human, as it might be put). So secular Humanism in the contemporary West is arguably undermined by Cultural Studies speculations about the 'post-human' because this is an *ontological* speculation – a 'cyborg' cannot reasonably be thought of as a member of any current biological species. Against this position it can be argued that it is highly misleading to claim that post-humans, even when defined as biological-machinic entities, presage an end to evolution and reduce secular institutions, values and reason to the illusory fashions of a pre-digital age.

I argue in this chapter that post-humanist concepts found in Cultural Studies antirealist and antiscientific writings offer no reason for rejecting either ethical or epistemological systems in which humans are regarded as central and unique. Indeed, I shall contend that 'Humanism', in its limited, 'scientific' sense, makes no assumptions about metaphysics at all: 'humans' are just one class of beings with certain characteristics that distinguish them as a species. Empirically, the more you know about the species' characteristics, the better you will be able to speculate and Theorize (or, better, theorize) about people as cultural agents, including their Cyborg potential and limitations.

Empirical psychology is necessarily species-specific, although that need not entail naïve evolutionary narratives or reductive neuro-physiological explanation. Like Schatzki, I want to resist 'a certain blackmail of the post-humanisms, namely that one is either a head-in-the-sand humanist or an up-to-date post-humanist' (Schatzki 2002: 194). Significantly, Cultural Studies' most popular ways of rejecting Humanism seem to be responses to this challenge. Theorists want to avoid falling into the head-in-the-sand camp, and instead wish to consider humans only in relation to their techno-cultural ecologies. So Schatzki quotes two writers much favoured by Cultural Studies commentators on science and psychological issues. Latour and Callon assert: 'Either we alternate between two absurdities (pure human world versus pure thing world – unenlightened humanism) or we redistribute actantial roles (attribute the properties of entities belonging to either world to entities of the other – clairvoyant humanism)' (Schatzki 2002: 194). Not a great choice: the naïve or the clairvoyant!

In the mainstream Cultural Studies literature, two Theorists have led the charge towards the horizon beyond which the human (as understood by Humanism) would be seen as a mirage of modernity, as passé because it was a construct of Enlightenment reason that resulted in rigid essentialism. Harraway (1991) and Hayles (1999a) examined the humanist world-view from an unlikely quarter. They emphasized the implications of Humanism for gender politics and liberation. Humanistic psychology and sociology were seen as essentialist, especially in regard to questions of gender. Their speculative techno-flesh entities are meant to provoke readers to ask whether current species concepts will be appropriate for describing the empirical entities that will 'become' after evolution ceases to obey the Darwinian rules formulated by last century's Science (itself an anachronism, perhaps). By implication, such ideas rework how 'we' [sic] think about old concerns like 'culture' or 'society', 'morality' or 'politics'.

Three principal overlapping sets of claims, speculations, or predictions about the actual or conceptual death of real human beings circulate in Cultural Studies. These can be sketched as follows:

1. Scientific advances will mean that human psychology will no longer be linked to particular human bodies, rendering obsolete the human individual understood as a corporeal entity. Minds will be downloaded into replaceable technologies to allow immortality of the subjective features of current members of the species. This is an alluring speculation, however much it sounds like a narcissistic Anglo-European fantasy (only about one fifth of the world's population currently has access to the Internet, so this fate is unlikely to befall many). Worse, the idea may not be logically, let alone physically, possible. Still, it has been predicted that by century's end, some humans will enjoy neural implants, their knowledge downloaded to computer memory: as Ray Kurtzweil (1999) speculates: '[T]heir identity will reside in software using replaceable nanobotic (cf. robotic) bodies as hardware.' If this leads to a significantly different human species, it would, as Searle puts it, presuppose 'evolution without DNA'.
2. Kurtzweil's speculation is an extreme version of the idea that the species is already being transformed unrecognizably by means of a series of technological prosthetic developments. Emerging machine-flesh entities will not be 'gendered', perhaps will not feel pain (and pleasure?), and so are not 'human' by definition. (This is Harraway's 'Cyborg' made manifest.) Bernardi presents Harraway's ideas thus: '[The] cyborg leads us towards a post-human world that is, by definition, post-gender, post-race, rich in abstraction … yet … fraught with socialist aspirations (Bernardi 2002: 157).' I am not sure how aspirations of any particular kind follow from merging flesh and machine but, leaving that aside, others share Harraway's idealization. Murphie and Potts (2003: 116) see the Cyborg as a way of imagining a world free of current gender 'demands and categories': 'The body will never be the body again' (Murphie & Potts 2003: 120). In short, the post-human is 'a contemporary exceeding [sic] of the human by entities thoroughly merged with machines' (2003: 28).
3. In other versions of this prediction, the emerging 'machines' may themselves be made of 'soft tissue'. Here, cryogenic suspension plus biological repair technologies will make flesh and blood people virtually immortal (or some of them at least). This speculation has radical implications for politics and morality, of course. (The film *Vanilla Sky*, Cameron Crowe 2001, plays with these.) Cloning and genetic engineering would eliminate inherited disease in this hopeful (or fearful) prediction. Again, evolution would presumably become passé. Humans (or once-were-humans) decide their own futures, transcending physical limitations.

Confusion reigns within Cultural Studies about which, if any, of these scenarios is possible or desirable, and about whether they are conceptual ideals or actual scientific predictions, so to speak. Perhaps predictably, Cultural Studies writing equivocates on these matters, but it does use the term 'post-human' to reject human*ism*, and to paint a future that it is hoped would be more politically correct because less gender- and race-torn than the present.

The more metaphysical or theoretically radical understanding of the post-Human found in Cultural Studies resorts to terms that I have already introduced, such as 'becoming'. However, the actual claims being made in this theoretical register are sometimes vague at best. Some writers seem content to show that, as 'nature is a Heraclitan fire' (as Gerard Manley Hopkins muses) and everything is in flux and 'becoming', the notion of biological species with actual qualities or defining characteristics is conceptually naïve (which seems to be the view of many commentators, including Colebrook (2002), discussed in earlier chapters).

Such writers have addressed the question of the post-human in purely verbal ways: for them, species talk is just a terminological preference doomed to obsolescence, perhaps like belief in the 'soul'. Their preference is phrased in terms of 'becoming' as a metaphor or actual process through which humans change, and is often linked to a utopian post-political anti-humanism. MacCormack (2008) sees Guatarri, for example, as proposing a 'refutation' of the concept of the hu-man [sic] insofar as it refers to the white male subject. (This would seem to beg the question, but I'll return to this problem later.) It is difficult to know what ontological status such a concept might have, as it appears to be simply a terminological preference. Hayles (1999a, 1999b) provides a similarly epistemologically vague account of the emergence of notions of the 'post-human', from computer/information systems to 'virtuality'. Yet it is unclear whether her account is meant to be read literally or 'literature-ly', so to speak. Certainly she shows how post-human*ist discourses* have developed through the twentieth-century displacement of physical by information paradigms such as cybernetic models of machines that can be thought of by analogy to human cognition. But the metaphorical and the empirical/realist claims of her analysis are difficult to disentangle.

Escaping the Human?

Other well-regarded Cultural Studies writers see the future of humans (as I will continue to call them) as somehow voluntary: 'Can humanity tweak itself into a new existence?' asks Massumi. And he answers in an odd, but revealing, way:

> The only way we will ever know is if the human collectivity applies itself to the development of the intervening technologies, which are then set up to sensitize and potentialize humanity-particles [sic] toward launching themselves instrumentally into their own futurity. By then, anyone (or anything) will no longer be human. (Massumi 2002: 123)

This would seem hard to argue against, although not for the reasons Massumi thinks. If his is typical of the way that Cultural Studies writers address analytically-difficult questions, then it is no surprise that students of this fast-disintegrating field are confused. In the new discourse, reified 'will' and 'desire' are given agency and a purely rhetorical, hence vacuous, analysis is presented. Typically, Massumi confuses empirical claims and predictions with merely terminological or definitional innovations lacking any precise empirical criteria for their application. It is hard to get the gist of what it means to be a 'humanity-particle' (or a collection of these, perhaps), a task not made any easier by being told that one's 'will' is unlikely to be 'relegated to adjacency and ... fully integrated into the [sic] transformative relay' (2002: 123). If nothing else, this kind of writing shows how difficult it is to be clear about what is at stake in claims about the post-human and to sort out the various kinds of claims currently being made around cyborgism, prosthetic augmentation and technologically-induced changes in 'subjectivity' to members of what we, at school, called the species *Homo sapiens*.

The prefix 'post-' is usually taken to mean 'after' or 'a new stage of' or 'an outgrowth of' the concept to which it is added. This makes it easy to understand that 'post-Elizabethan' refers to the period after that Queen's reign. But in the case of concepts with complex reference, such as 'human', matters are more difficult. So in trying to enter into debate with Theorists who make claims about the nature, or causes, of post-humanity, one seeks for (or perhaps assumes) a definition of the *essential characteristics* that license the use of the original term. What might 'human' mean if the late Christopher Reeve or *The Terminator* (James Cameron, 1984) or Deckard, in *Blade Runner* (Ridley Scott, 1982), is said to be 'after' or 'beyond' human? If the claim is made that the species is being altered by actual technologically-mediated extensions that change 'subjectivity', then one is entitled to ask: what exactly are these revolutionary or evolutionary alterations to the species?

Answers to these kinds of questions can only be given if one stipulates some necessary (not just incidental or accompanying) qualities of those flesh-and-blood entities that populate the globe and are, in fact, members of the same species. Clearly, this raises the need for a precise definition of 'species'. For if post-human speculations are meaningful, they must imply at least something empirical about the transformation of the species into a new species – that is, a new biological class with new defining characteristics. Or, a stronger claim might be at stake – something like the proposition that the very idea of species will melt away. A new vocabulary to describe the 'beyond human' phenomena will emerge, one that gradually replaces the old terminology. For example, if one defining characteristic of a species is that it is an interbreeding group of organisms that produces fertile offspring, then technologically-enhanced 'replicants', cyborgs, or some such, might reproduce non-biologically and/or even be immortal yet still be classified as members of the original species. In both cases – the weaker and the stronger – coherent argument presupposes a definition of 'human' and 'species' with which to debate the competing claims.

Despite Massumi's optimism, it seems unlikely that people will decide to 'launch' voluntarily whatever the changes might be that characterize his revolutionary 'futurity', especially if they have no way of describing their existing qualities as a species (Massumi might refer to this as their 'previousness'). (As an aside, I cannot resist commenting that the literature on this issue makes it hard to repress a Gary Larson-like image of a group of chimpanzees sitting in a circle planning for their progeny to visit Disneyland after undergoing the necessary collectively-willed species-modification into humanoids.)

Unfortunately, much of the most abstract and ambiguous writing in English about the post-Human endorses the peculiar metaphysics of Deleuze that I have already discussed in other contexts. This post-structuralist orientation leads to the postulation of 'becomings' rather than old-fashioned entities as the fundamental furniture of the universe. To see how this ontology underpins the oddly immaterial enterprise, let me quote Colebrook's version of generic 'post-structuralism':

> Post-structuralists in general rejected the idea that we could examine a static structure of differences [sic] that might give us some point of foundation for knowing the world. Post-structuralism sought to explain [sic] the emergence, becoming or genesis of structures: ... for this reason, Deleuze and those of his generation sought to conceptualise both difference and becoming, but a difference and becoming that would not be the becoming of some being.

It should be noted that Colebrook writes of a 'foundation for knowing the world', even though the world is not made up of situations, objects, or 'beings'. Massumi's version of post-structuralism also seems content to omit objects, beings or 'things', in favour of agent-less verb-processes made into nouns, such as 'becomings'. Yet this assumption is used to elevate (or to reduce) materiality to dynamic processes with which to think a 'virtual' realm: 'life', according to Colebrook's version of Deleuze, is a 'virtual power to become', but not towards some already 'given' end, or on the basis of what already exists (Colebrook 2002). Humans, being a form of life, would be part of this peculiarly non-teleological teleology. But, leaving this aside, Massumi presents a similarly romantic phenomenology that reaffirms what might be seen as a kind of voluntarism: 'Desire is the condition of evolution.' Does this mean that 'desire' is a necessary, or even sufficient, condition for evolutionary change? In either case, what is changing? It cannot be the 'becomings' themselves, so it must be the species (the gene pool that currently defines a species) that is being transformed. Without further linguistic self-flagellation, I think we are justified in concluding that writing about 'becomings' in the abstract will not tell us much about what 'post-humanity' might actually involve. It is a mere tautology in Deleuze-speak. Let me therefore move from 'becoming-Human' to the tantalizing notion of the 'trans-human'.

Posting a series of utopian speculations on the Internet under this heading is a writer ('strategic futurist' or 'strategic philosopher') known as Max More (1994). Somewhat predictably citing Nietzsche, More hopes to 'overcome' man by becoming 'posthuman' (no need for hyphens in this popularized version of the theme). He accuses many Humanists of being afraid of 'their own promethean urge to challenge the gods' and so unambiguously proclaims his romantic desires. Less tentative than Hayles or Massumi, More waxes enthusiastic about actual post-human futures, using the abstract language of 'new age' psychology to publicize his 'Extropian' goals:

> Extropians have a specific conception of transhumanism, involving certain values and goals, such as boundless expansion, self-transcendence, dynamic optimism, intelligent technology, and spontaneous order. Extropians are those who consciously seek to further 'extropy', a measure of intelligence, information, energy, life, experience, diversity, opportunity, and growth. (More 1994: np)

He goes on to cite current scientific developments as harbingers of these utopian (or narcissistic) enthusiasms:

> Yet we should regard transhuman transcendence as natural. Nature embodies within itself a tendency to seek new complex structures, to overcome itself to take on new, more effective forms. Nietzsche recognized this in his view of the universal will to power. More recently, we have partly uncovered this drive towards complexity through complexity theory, evolutionary theory, artificial life, and neurocomputing. Overcoming limits comes naturally to humans. The drive to transform ourselves and our environment is at our core. (More 1994: np)

Note that, like the abstracted notion of 'becomings', this advertisement for our 'core' presupposes its own very specific model of 'human nature'. The pseudo-scientific vocabulary of 'complexity theory' and computing is invoked to justify More's wishful promethean unboundedness. He encourages his readers to follow him on his speculative journey by asking us to ignore the punitive superego that holds them back: 'No-one will punish us for opening Pandora's box, for equipping ourselves with wings of posthuman intelligence and agelessness' (1994: np).

Although this can be seen as a rather infantile version of the wish to transcend one's mortality and other corporeal limitations by means of actual technological augmentation or by theoretical abstraction, More's invocations are typical of the means also cited by more circumspect writers. Indeed, they echo the kinds of technologies cited by Harraway and Hayles, whose cyborgs and post-humans, of course, though not seen purely in the future tense, are similarly utopian. In a related vein (if I may use a pun), Massumi (2002) has written at length about what he sees as the philosophical significance of the 'body artist' known as Stelarc, claiming that 'the end of evolution is at hand', no less. Additionally, in their Media Studies textbook, Murphie and Potts (2003) also invoke Stelarc as a focal example in their discussion of cyborgs. However, they note (*pace* Massumi 2002: 110) that the cyborg is a metaphor or a metonym for emerging forms of cyber-mediated social relations/interactions, rather than an entity displacing members of the species as presently configured. But if one regards social relations as necessary to the definition of humans qua humans, then the use of the cyborg to 'imagine a world free of gender demands and categories' renders humans as we think we know them things of the past. No gendered social relations, to put the matter crudely, no *homo sapiens*. The technologically-augmented humanoid might be seen as post-human precisely because it is post-gender and post-social. But in the absence of any clear idea of what *defines* the species, it is hard to pin down the implications of such speculations.

Murphie and Potts do claim some positive qualities for their emerging hybrid, however: 'If we ask what the body wants, the answer today is that it wants more information' (2003: 120). But, surely, information is only information in relation to pre-given needs or specific social contexts. I cannot really understand what it means to say a machine or a species 'wants information' in the abstract. Can any such entity 'want' as opposed to *need* information in the usual senses of these terms?

The reification of the concept of 'information' in these discussions, plus the attribution of motives and drives to emerging post-Humans, are clearly meant to be rhetorical rather than literal claims about any actual class of entities. Yet, the epistemological status of these claims is unclear. Although they call it a 'metaphor', Murphie and Potts at times revert to a more literal discussion of the cyborg and reiterate some of the confusions or equivocations that beset Cultural Studies speculations, including Hayles's discussion of the post-human. Like her, they speak of the 'body' and of 'embodiment', but end by claiming that bodies are, or at least can be thought of as, 'forms of information interacting with other forms of information, or as patterns of randomness interacting with other patterns of randomness, tearing patterns apart, creating or perceiving new patterns' (Murphie & Potts 2003: 129). So the post-human seems to be a 'contemporary exceeding of the human by entities thoroughly merged with machines' (2003: 28). Note that in this context the 'post-' prefix is not meant to be interpreted as temporal. Rather it refers to 'more than' or an 'exceeding' of the human – as currently defined, I assume. So the kinds of changes or 'exceedings' that variously carry the prefix 'post-' in this sense can be difficult to describe precisely:

> This mutant, posthuman is not a matter of armoring the body, adding robotic prostheses, or technologically transferring consciousness from the body; it is not, in other words, a matter of fortifying the boundaries of the subject, of acknowledging the relations and mutational processes that constitute it. A posthuman subject position [note the shift] would in other words, acknowledge the otherness that is part of us. It would involve opening boundaries of individual and collective identity, changing the relations that have distinguished between the subject and the object, self and others, us and them. (Rutsky 1999: 21–2)

This is a very vague claim. It rejects the more empirical proposals made by most other commentators. By retreating to the now-familiar abstraction of 'the subject position', it reads as neither biological nor technological. But why label the concept 'mutant' or 'post-Human' at all, unless this is simply to show that the author considers current humans also to be merely 'subject positions', albeit ones of which he does not sound very fond?

Problems of Coherence

I hope I have shown that the literature on 'the post-human' concept moves from utopian, transcendental hopes to abstracted notions of 'information' and 'becomings', the latter sometimes given empirical definition. Some writers resort to the most vague of terms, such as semiotic 'subject positions' to designate what is at stake. However, the 'weaker' versions do not seem to offer much advance on the stronger, more empirical analyses, other than to obfuscate them.

Second, the literature often insinuates the concept of 'post-humanity' into arguments about the overthrow of the episteme (the conventional knowledge paradigm), so undermining the ethics of post-Enlightenment, secular 'human*ism*'. It is not always clear how the two are relevant to each other, as I have mentioned. Additionally, the literature is unclear about whether computers are causing the species (or its 'subjectivity', its psychology?) to change unrecognizably, or whether computers and digitization, web cultures, etc. merely provide metaphors, analogies and homologies by which to understand how people think and feel because of how they are enmeshed in the ever-changing ecologies of technology.

As this whistle-stop tour has been a bumpy ride, let me conclude by recapping the most patent methodological problems that beset the post-human literature of Cultural Studies:

1. Theorists' failure to define specifically any qualities or characteristics of humans which would be changed in ways that implied how the species would change. (My working definition of a species would be: 'an inter-breeding, mortal population with innate qualities ecologically attuned to its environment of adaptedness'.)
2. Equivocation, evident in concepts that move many of the commentaries from empirical speculations to idealist and vague wishes about 'becoming other' – other than what? In what respects or aspects? One might ask.
3. Vagueness about what class of entities is being transformed. This allows commentators to evade saying just what the mechanisms could mediate or effect change: for instance, dubious processes like 'downloads' of mental phenomena, the concept of the species as 'information-driven' and defined – these are not detailed enough to suggest what kinds of changes are empirically possible or likely.
4. Even the logical possibilities about which the debate swirls are occluded by conceptual naïveté, especially reification of concepts and of relations. This amounts to endorsing a non-realist epistemology because 'any theory that denies a realist (non-constitutive) theory of relations and denies that statements can unambiguously refer to states of affairs [is non-realist]' (Hibberd 2001: 343); and 'a relation can only be meaningfully spoken of as holding between two independent terms'(2001: 395). In short, the failure to

independently define both the species that is to 'become' and the entities it will become reduces the relational term 'becomings' (itself a curious reification) to little more than rhetoric.

Recall that Colebrook (Chapters 1 & 2) renders metaphysical just such empirical phenomena via 'becomings':

> Post-structuralists, in general, rejected the idea that we could examine a static structure of differences that might give us some point of foundation for knowing the world. Post-structuralism sought to explain the emergence, becoming or genesis of structures ... For this reason, Deleuze and those of his generation sought to conceptualise both difference and becoming, but a difference and becoming that would not be the becoming of some being. (Colebrook 2002: 3)

Clearly, this is a despairing epistemology, one in which all knowable entities, including the human species, simply evaporate.

Despite these problems, Hayles has raised the stakes in the debate by writing that 'the emergence of the post-human as an informational material entity is paralleled by a corresponding reinterpretation of the deep structure of the physical world' (Hayles 1999b: 11). This seems to give a material status to the notion of the 'post-human', regarding it as part of a revolution in the physical sciences. But is she really pretending that Cultural Studies has revolutionized metaphysics with its neo-ontology of 'becomings'? Perhaps what she means is that the speculations are consistent with new notions of genetics and gene expression, with changed definitions of information, as it is understood in cybernetics, etc. Despite Deleuze, Massumi et al, it remains to be demonstrated that humanities writers have contributed conceptual clarity about, let alone any new evidence relevant to, any particular 'reinterpretation of the deep structure of the physical world'. Worse, to make this sweeping claim, Hayles assumes that humans were not previously thought of as 'informational material' – which seems particularly odd given that Psychology has always studied both physiology and cognition and what Theorists might call their 'co-instantiation'.

Hayles's confusions multiply when she contests the putative separation of 'materiality' from 'information', seeming content to see 'information ... as pattern', and hence not tied to any particular material instantiation, but 'free to travel across time and space' (Hayles 1999b: 12). This way of speaking may just mean that information can be recoded and transmitted in many material forms, but that is hardly an ontological revolution. So it is difficult to see what is being claimed when writers personify terms like 'information' and claim, for instance, that it 'wants to be free'. Yet she does set limits on the motivations of information, and accepts that even if 'we become the information we have constructed we can(not) achieve immortality'. And she allows that 'for information to exist [*sic*], it must *always* be instantiated in a medium' (1999b; 13). Equivocation indeed!

I have discussed this analysis in detail to show that the rhetorical, especially the metaphorical, style of such writing can lead to inconsistencies and conceptual slippages that make its claims difficult to evaluate at best. Worse, they leave the reader with the uneasy feeling that the claims made are banal, self-contradictory or logically incoherent. Certainly they would surprise experts in the biological and physical, not to mention the psychological, sciences.

Like science fiction generally, post-human speculations present hypothetico-deductive experiments: they speculate about what would happen if one or more feature of the current species were changed or eliminated. The science fiction genre narrativizes much the same conceptual experiments. For example, the film *Zardoz* (John Boorman 1974) speculated on what humans would become if they were immortal, and many novels and films explore the plausible consequences of a humanity consisting of only one gender in which males have become redundant. Perhaps the principal difference between science fiction films and Cultural Studies writing on the concept of the post-human is that the former are generally dystopian and realist-humanist whereas the latter is generally utopian, epistemologically idealist and anti-humanist. Like most of my students, I would trust the ontologically responsible films rather than the capital-T Theorists, at least on matters of psychology and sociology.

Post-human concepts and post-humanist speculation may have appealed to Theorists because they promise a utopia where technology allows people to transcend their genetic imperfections and limitations, overcoming also the politics of gender binaries. Whatever the motives, however, the post-human ideal does not seem to offer students useful ways to escape the dilemmas that arise when they try to understand people – either as physical objects or as continuously changing subjects. This is because, in order coherently to discuss *actual species* and *real psychological change*, we must, at some stage in our debates, *attribute qualities to classes of entities*. We must, to put it bluntly, predicate something of something. This is true whether the entities are designed by Hollywood, by Dr Frankenstein, or whether they are the conceptual inventions of Cultural Studies Theorists.

Chapter 6

Affecting Ontologies

We have first raised a dust then complain we cannot see.
George Berkeley

This is a powerful crayon: It's got power in it.
Zara Podmore, aged 5

Affect as an Entity

To judge a poem as 'lively' or a musical performance 'arresting' or 'affecting' is to say something about one's response to it. Such responses are, obviously, psychological and refer to the sensations and meanings that the respective cultural work evokes in the listener/viewer. More precisely, aesthetic talk refers to sensing, perceiving and interpreting *in relation to* the work to which the person is responding, a point that Theorists might endorse. Of course, individual responses will depend on the audience member's particular history of exposure to, and knowledge of, the aesthetic/cultural field in which the new experience is situated. Unsurprisingly, Cultural Studies aims to describe and to analyse these experiences and the various ways by which people speak about them. It is concerned with aesthetics and culture in the general sense discussed in previous chapters, so it discusses psychological responses to sensory-aesthetic stimulation and to meaningful 'texts'. Famous examples of Cultural Studies writing about psychological responses to 'texts' range from Roland Barthes's eloquent ruminations on his late mother's photograph to Ien Ang's interpretations of why women viewers enjoyed the soap opera *Dallas*.

When used in English as a noun, 'affect' is synonymous with 'feeling', or sometimes 'emotion'. Obsolete usage suggests some of the connotations that cling to the term today: affection (amorous feelings), passion and general sensation. Psychologists describe people who are unemotional as 'lacking affect', and also refer to 'inappropriate affect', for example when people laugh at others' suffering or their own pain. Freud's psychology is replete with references to 'affect'. In *The Interpretation of Dreams*, he uses the term principally to refer to changes in the experience of pleasure or 'unpleasure' within an economy of 'psychical energy': 'The pleasure of humour ... comes about – we cannot say otherwise – at the cost of a release of affect that does not occur: it arises from *an economy in the expenditure of affect*' (Freud 1976: 293, emphasis added).

Notice that for Freud, affect involves the feeling of pleasure and its opposite, and is developed within a generally homeostatic or economic model of drives (instincts). The motivational basis of his analysis of humour assumes that people are hedonistic – driven to seek pleasure and to avoid pain, both psychological and physical. The precursors to Freud's notion of the concept of 'affect' and to his and William James' analyses of its relation to cognition are widely discussed in the psycho-philosophical literature, for example by Redding (1999). However, recent Cultural Studies writers have more or less ignored Freud's hedonistic assumption, preferring to take up Deleuze's more metaphysical use of the term, derived instead from Spinoza.

The one word can, of course, be used to refer to more than one 'concept', and Deleuze's 'affect' differs radically from Freud's, as it does from everyday English interpretations (as we shall see presently). However, in Spinoza's monistic metaphysics, 'affectus' is usually translated as 'emotion' in English (e.g. Monk & Raphael, 2001). Moreover, it carries more active, almost *causal* connotations in Spinoza (*Ethics*, Part 3, 1677), connotations which are echoed in some Cultural Studies writing that seeks to move beyond motivational psychology by invoking 'affect' as a kind of general 'force' and even as a condition of the *physical* world in general. That is, affect is seen as more than a realist bio-psychological phenomenon in many cultural/aesthetic contexts especially, a point I will develop in this chapter. I will consider how Cultural Studies commentators borrowing from Deleuze have erected an all-purpose psycho-aesthetic concept with which to describe willy-nilly a multitude of reactions to works of art, and have then extended the application of this term to try to describe the works themselves. Thus, not content to postulate 'affect' in *people* responding to the perceptible world, including artworks, commentators attribute 'affect' to the material world itself, where it serves a number of strangely animistic purposes, as I will illustrate.

The concept of 'affect' has intruded into earlier chapters. Here I wish to consider it more fully in terms of its implications for causal accounts of psychological phenomena and for the more general question of what philosophers of science call 'vitalism' – the postulation of 'inner forces' as unseen causes. Vitalism involves the positing and reifying of energies, unobservable qualities, and abstract words as causally relevant to changes in animate and even in inanimate phenomena – hence the amusing example of my five-year-old friend, Zara, who attributed 'power' to her perfectly ordinary crayon. Like vitalists generally, Zara assumes an unseen 'level of reality' and postulates a magical causal power to explain why her crayon works as it does. (Of course, I do not wish to criticize my five-year-old ontologist for naïvety, merely to note the similarity between her postulations and those of many sophisticated Theory writers.)

In Cultural Studies, as in religion, the verbal creation of a world of pulsating micro-forces allows writers to continually poeticize mundane matters of experience such as perception, and to write about what sound like new kinds of aesthetics and science. To the vitalist, objective science is not enough: the world of cultural responsiveness must involve 'excess' (of something, though it is not always clear exactly what). What are today called the 'Life Sciences' are restricted to what Massumi calls 'dumb matter'. Science misses the vital, the life forces, the shimmering 'affect' that animates the universe, at least according to the most egregious examples of Theory's speculative attacks on realist approaches to studying bio-psychological phenomena. 'Power', 'intensity', 'affect', and other reifications pepper the Theory texts that Cultural Studies presents in its sometimes mystifying curriculum.

For many students, the term 'affect' found its way into Cultural Studies via Deleuze's highly influential aesthetics/psychology of cinema, published in English as *Cinema One/Two*. Writing about the way in which films address and affect actual audiences obliged Deleuze to revert to the language of real phenomena and real people. He only sporadically assumes his 'process' ontology of 'becomings' rather than material 'things' and events (to put the matter in terms I have had to employ in Chapter 2). Briefly, this means that the methodologies of his books on cinema are more conventional than those of his metaphysically-focused writing. So objects, images, and films at least serve as grammatical subjects of empirical propositions, even if his phenomenological and objective styles of analysis frequently overlap. For example, discussing images of faces (including 'close-ups'), he speaks of 'features' of faces, of actual represented parts of the body etc., in conventionally 'realist' ways.

Students who have only encountered concepts like 'affect' in Deleuze's cinema writing nevertheless face many of the epistemological difficulties that confront them in his more metaphysical works. He adopts a phenomenologically inventive style that seldom clearly indicates whether the concepts he employs are psychological (describe people's experiences) or are semiotic (describe aspects of cinematic representation per se). So *Cinema One* confounds many readers unused to descriptions of phenomenological processes, albeit rendered in deceptively empirical terms. In a chapter discussing 'The Affect as Entity', for example, Deleuze elaborates and abstracts the psychological processes that he thinks are involved in seeing images of faces. He speaks of 'Powers', 'Qualities' and 'Icons' [sic]. These are given partial definition in his idiosyncratic way, but they are also linked to common psychological predicates – 'sensation, sentiment, emotion or even impulse (*pulsion*) in a person'. The general concept that organizes his highly wrought analyses is the 'affection-image':

> There are affects of things. The edge, the blade, or rather 'the point' of Jack the Ripper's knife, is no less an affect than the fear which overcomes his features and the whole of his face. (Deleuze 1986: 97)

'Affect' here seems to reside 'in' the audience responding to the image, but also in the quality of the actor's expressions ('the fear ...'). This is confusing at best. If audiences in the cinema feel some emotion when they see a knife's blade, then the 'affect', surely, is part of their response that is culturally 'coded'. Whether an image provokes affect is contingent on the 'meanings' that the depicted objects have in their cultural contexts. Maybe some facial expressions also evoke particular *innate* emotional responses such as anxiety, but whether this occurred in particular cases would be an empirical question.

Deleuze trades on the various ambiguities of his psychological-sounding concepts: are they attributes of images or responses 'in' people? Are they psychological or semiotic concepts? Are they innate and universal, or conventional and particular? Are they learned when we go to the cinema to see images and observe people's behaviours and expressions? Unfortunately, Deleuze is unconcerned with such questions. Instead he writes about what I would call the emotional impact of seeing faces and representations of face-like phenomena by means of a relay of abstract terms:

> The affect is the entity, that is Power or Quality. It is something expressed: the affect does not exist independently of something which expresses it, although it is completely

> distinct from it. What expresses it is a face or a facial equivalent (a faceified object) or, as we will see later, even a proposition. We call the set of the expressed and its expression, of the affect and the face, 'icon' … The affection-image is power or quality considered for themselves, as expressed. It is clear [*sic*] that powers and qualities can also exist in a completely different way: as actualised, embodied in states of things. (Deleuze 1986: 97)

More definitional chains lead to several more or less empirical, mundane propositions:

> In a state of things which actualises them the quality becomes the 'quale' of an object, power becomes action or passion, affect becomes sensation, sentiment, emotion or even impulse (pulsion) in a person, the face becomes the character or mask of the person (it is only from this point of view that there can be mendacious expressions). But we are no longer in the domain of the affection-image, we are in the domain of the action-image. (Deleuze 1986: 97)

Therefore, it is asserted, faces and images of faces affect people (or, perhaps, evoke 'affect'). But Deleuze cannot resist the temptation to render as metaphysical even this most banal psychological observation. He creates reified 'concepts' that seem to reveal dimensions of reality ('pulsions', 'emotions', 'powers' and 'qualities') by no more than the expedient of word-magic. Affect (as entity) seems to be and to do many things. It is attributed causal efficacy, as in:

> The affection-image … is abstracted from the spatio-temporal coordinates which would relate it to a state of things, and abstracts the face from the person to which it belongs in the state of things. (Deleuze, 1986: 97)

So the 'affects of things' (above) are no more than the connotations of the things and/or their representation, as determined by cultural agreement. The 'affect' of the edge of a knife surely is no more (or less) than how it provokes emotional (or affective) experience in cinema audiences. There is simply no need to posit an all-purpose 'affect', or to assume that examining the cinema reveals a new class of phenomena called 'affection-images', which somehow exist independently of 'states of things'. Like young Zara's discussion of her crayon's powers, this analysis is purely verbal – it re-states the phenomena as its own explanation, so to speak. This way of writing means there is no end to the concepts that might be postulated because no independent evidence can be offered for their referents.

As the example of 'affect' shows, not all words name useful 'concepts'. Words can be used to refer to situations or things in the world only when people are in general agreement that they do, and when their respective referents can be inferred by means of inter-subjectively reliable observation. Verbal inventiveness and reification, attributing powers to affects and images (or their combined effect) does not illuminate the way in which people respond to images on the silver screen or anywhere else. Defining one's terms may be a necessary aspect of psychological and aesthetic analysis, but it is not sufficient. Worse, in the affect-faciality analysis Deleuze seems to be 'making it up as he goes along', to use a colloquialism.

Despite the dubious value of the concept, 'affect' is ubiquitous in Cultural Studies and film studies writing where its provenance is usually Deleuzian. However, it is not used in a methodologically rigorous way to designate psychological or psycho-physiological events, despite or because of its theoretical adaptability. For example, Colebrook glosses the term thus:

> Affects are sensible experiences in their singularity liberated from organising systems of representations ... Affect, as presented in art, disrupts the everyday and opinionated [sic] links we make between words and experience. (2002: 22–3)

Other authors writing about the way in which people experience temporal aspects of cinema invoke the same term and also claim it as Deleuzian, albeit in vague ways. They may insist that it does *not* refer to 'emotion', but assert that

> [c]inema becomes the means to experience time as effectively charged with anxiety, pleasure, trauma and desire ... affect is a very specific term [sic] that registers the psychological effects of time on both the spectating and performing body ... affect, or more particularly an affective experience of time [sic] allows for an identification of the specificity of bodily responses to filmic movement. (Rassos 2006: 2–3)

Such a non-emotional response to abstract time is nothing if not elusive. Confusing even, especially when the writer also postulates 'affects' in the plural being 'generated by films'. The writer cites Deleuze and Guattari's adaptation of Spinoza's 'affectus' in their book *A Thousand Plateaus: Capitalism and Schizophrenia*, where, Rassos tells us, 'affect' 'is characterized as 'an ability to affect and be affected'. The French philosophers go on to suggest that a real effect can be attributed to 'affective responsiveness': it allows the body to move from 'one experiential state ... to another ... implying an augmentation or diminution in that body's capacity to act' (Rassos 2006, p. 3).

So a distinctly psychological-sounding word is invoked to cover a complex series of actual psychological-cum-physiological processes, it seems. But 'affect' is just one term used by Cultural Studies in its attempt to found a conceptually-new understanding of people and culture. I have indicated how terms with multiple but vague definition, terms which may refer to no observable or potentially observable phenomena, can be created as causally effective, but only in facile and quite arbitrary ways. When this is done, a kind of unseen animating force can be postulated, something that lives 'deep down things' (to quote from the romantic Jesuit poet, Gerard Manley Hopkins). Sometimes the postulated process is so vague as to be of no analytical value (as in 'the ability to affect and to be affected', above). Other metaphysically-odd terms can also be invoked for rhetorical effect. One that stands out in relation to psychological forces of a Deleuzian kind is 'quasi-causality'. Massumi writes that:

> Quasi-causality concerns something very different (from causality): practically absent material potential. A potential does not pre-exist its emergence [sic]. If it doesn't emerge, it's because it wasn't really there. If it does it really just arrives. Potential is an advent ... Surprise. Matter boost. In effect, uncaused. Self-creative activity in and of the world. (Massumi 2002: 226)

This sounds at best like a series of metaphors or rhetorical moves designed to evoke a sense of wonder at the how the world works (or, perhaps, at Massumi's ability to juggle words in unconventional ways). Yet Massumi uses this kind of writing to advance his rejection of conventional psychology and biology. He writes as though it were axiomatic that what he labels 'science' cannot deal with 'the virtual' and 'the emergent' (used as nouns, not adjectives). Science is deaf to the 'self-creative activity in and of the world'. To open one's ears, one needs 'Philosophy' (with a capital P):

> Philosophy operates at the imminent limit of science, 'downstream' of its beginning terminus in recognisability, approaching nature's of-itself. What operates beyond science's outside limit, its end terminus in reproducibility? This is the empirical region of quality, understood as the actual expression of virtuality or relationality. (Massumi, 2002: 248)

A great deal seems to be happening in the fluid quasi-causal world where 'better-than-science' Cultural Studies concepts are coined and given currency. The sceptical student, on the other hand, might be inclined to agree with the psychologist John Maze, who argues that realism demands commitment to a coherent use of language:

> Realism founds itself ... on the requirements of coherent, intelligible discourse. One of these with wide ramifications is the rejection of the concept of intrinsic or constitutive relations, that is, the notion that an entity can have its relations intrinsic to its own nature without any correlative terminus. A relation can only be meaningfully spoken of as holding between two independent terms (Maze 2001: 395).

Many of Massumi's concepts are of the kind that Maze rejects: postulations that attribute material reality to relations as such. Worse, 'relationality' is seen as an entity that has qualities in itself! In Anglophone philosophy, such concepts are usually said to be reified when they are used as though they refer to material entities. Like the other writers quoted above, Massumi trades on the ambiguity of the grammatical status of his terminology to describe the in- or un-describable. He reifies terms and then claims they are 'infra-empirical' after all. And he has his followers, although they usually limit their borrowings to the all-purpose 'affect'.

The prominent geographer Nigel Thrift (2004) 'attempts to take the politics of affect as not just incidental but central to the life of cities ... consider[ing] the systematic engineering of affect'. However, despite his commendation of Massumi, Thrift vacillates between defining 'affect' as 'emotion(s)' (à la Darwin, he suggests), and understanding it 'as a form of thinking, often indirect and non-reflective, it is true, but thinking all the same' and also 'as a set of embodied practices that produce visible conduct as an outer lining'. As the quote suggests, this is not so much a concept as a complete socio-psychology, all performed by a single word! Like Massumi, Thrift seems to embrace phenomenology as the royal road to the material, 'to develop descriptions of how emotions occur in everyday life, understood as the richly expressive/aesthetic feeling-cum-behaviour of continual becoming that is provided chiefly by bodily states and processes (and which are understood as constitutive of affect)' (Thrift 2004: 4).

As we have seen in Deleuze and Massumi, in this case 'becoming' seems to be an ontologically slippery kind of process, and 'affect' a factotum reification. Thrift persists in assuming that the feelings of vitality that accompany or constitute (?) the 'doing of emotions' are 'a kind of metamorphosis' (2004: 4). Again, Cultural Studies displaces social science via phenomenology to postulate actual psycho-physiological processes. What else could 'affect' refer to? Thrift goes on to talk about 'neuropolitics' and quotes William Connolly, another highly regarded Cultural Studies academic: 'the dense series of counterloops among cinema, TV, philosophy, neurophysiology and everyday life ... mean that we do not recognize the realm between thinking and affects' (Thrift 2004: 69). It is tempting to say that I, for one, certainly do not recognize this realm.

As a result of his paradoxical phenomenology of the unnoticed realm between thinking and affect, Thrift comes to an ontologically definite conclusion: 'There is more to the world than is routinely acknowledged ... and this excess is not just incidental' (2004: 72). 'Excess' is another of the terms that infect Cultural Studies discourse. It works rather like 'affect' or 'virtuality' – a vitalist 'beyond the limits of science' kind of word: another 'big mysterious extra ingredient in all living things' that seems always to evade precise specification', to quote Daniel Dennett (2005: 78).

Thrift's invocation of what I see as the vitalist concept of 'affect' is approvingly taken up in other Cultural Studies online journals such as *Ephemera: theory and politics in organization*. In a section titled 'Moving Minds, or What is Politics?' Jordan Crandall presents a more detailed gloss of Deleuzian 'affect', and alludes to Thrift in the process:

According to Deleuze, affect fills the interval between perception and action. It is a modality of perceptions that ceases to yield an action and instead brings forth an expression. It is not about movement, but rather the quality of a lived interior state, which marks a pure coincidence between subject and object. It is a movement that is not engaged outwardly but absorbed inwardly – a tendency or interior effort that halts just this side of doing. It is about how one experiences oneself as oneself from the inside ... It is the perception of one's aliveness, vitality, and changeability, which can be seen as 'freedom' ... It is about the incorporealization of information, not its representation: a corporeal thinking that is preconscious and pre-active, and which does not resolve to a statement.

As Nigel Thrift suggests, this is a site that has become increasingly analysable and explicitly political through practices and techniques aimed at it specifically ... measurable through new technologies of tracking and filtering that are able to probe into the intimate and nearly instantaneous states of bodily movement, orientation, disposition, mood, arrayed as calculations, statistics, cross-referenced with database records of consumer or citizen behaviour: a newly constituted body of measurable states and functions, whose inclinations to act are quantifiable and understood as predictable. (Crandall 2005: 760)

What is most confusing here is the apparent definition of terms by proliferating other terms that are themselves undefined, and the willy-nilly postulation of all manner of processes, events, entities, and states. Recalling Chapters 3 and 4, notice also that the 'subject' is 'coincidental with the object' when 'affect' fills the interval between perception and action. No less noteworthy is the risible claim to scientific methodological sophistication concerning ways of 'measuring' 'inclinations to act'. Crandall tries to exemplify the manifestations of these micro-psychological processes, however, by citing what seems like a banal observable indication of his elaborate concepts:

According to John Armitage, the US Department of Homeland Security's 'Be Ready' campaign operates on this space of imminent mobility. The readiness it promotes has no real object, and is simply in a kind of self-generating machine ... Desire and fear cohabit here at the threshold of action. (Crandall 2005)

Just why the term 'political' is used in this context is difficult to discern. Crandall suggests that consumer behaviour functions as a mock freedom, giving 'both pleasure and defence', although this prosaic insight seems conceptually independent of the 'affect' he invokes. The notion that Deleuzian vitalism is relevant to 'politics', however, echoes throughout other recent Cultural Studies and post-disciplinary writing, to which I now return.

The Trinity: Feeling, Emotion, Affect

We have seen how the term 'affect' is used in an essentially psychological way, even though it seems to refer to no particular kind of psychological process. Some Cultural Studies commentators, however, have tried to describe 'affect' in more realist ways – Shouse, for example – who also cites Deleuze and Massumi as his guide:

Affect is non-conscious experience [sic] of intensity; it is a moment of unformed or unstructured potential. Affect is always prior to and outside of language ... because it is always prior to and outside of consciousness ... Affect is the body's way of preparing itself for action ... [T]he body doesn't just absorb pulses or discrete stimulation, it infolds contexts. (Massumi, 2002: 30 quoted in Shouse, 2005: np)

Nevertheless, the 'affect' of this passage still sounds like a concept as unnecessary as it is surprising. But at least Shouse thinks that something actually happens in real bodies, however much this pushes him into reifications that even his mentor might doubt:

Without affect, feelings do not 'feel' because they have no intensity ... [A]ffect plays an important part in determining the relationship between our bodies, our environment, and others, and the subjective experience we feel/think as affect dissolves into experience. (Shouse 2005: np)

Shouse goes on to agree with Massumi that this non-conscious experience acts as 'affection', 'the process whereby affect is transmitted between bodies'. On Shouse's account, feelings, emotions and affect (not affects) are distinct, the last being 'what determines the intensity (quantity) of a feeling (quality), as well as the background intensity of our everyday lives (the half-sensed ongoing hum of quantity/quality we experience when we are not really attuned to any experience at all).'

Therefore, the attempt to make the concept refer to some actual process becomes utterly confusing. This results from reifying 'intensity' and 'quantity'. The most charitable interpretation of the postulated 'affect' and 'affectus' that I can offer is to see them as referring to something like 'arousal', 'liveliness' or 'responsiveness', although this renders them of little 'scientific' value. Another way of understanding such concepts is to say they are, at best, epiphenomenal – like the shadow of an object, so to speak, not materially relevant to understanding physical processes, but merely an 'accompanying' incidental aspect of the phenomenon in question. However, Massumi and his followers do not see 'affect' as epiphenomenal; instead, they insist on its reality, claiming that it acts as a causal factor in many contexts. In effect, they infer it from what Massumi calls his 'hyperrealism' (!)

I have argued that these all-too-typical ways of writing about human culture reject the claims of social and psychological science as naïvely positivistic and/or realist. They postulate a 'crowd' of concepts (or words at least) that evoke a vitalist realm beyond science, beyond observation. I have presented some examples of renowned Cultural Studies writers who fondly cite each other's concepts to support a curiously vitalist ontology. Massumi, Connolly and Thrift are not isolated cases. What makes critiquing these modes of writing practically impossible, however, is the fact that the idealist concepts that furnish their universes are simply *assumed* to be meaningful, and are given no explicit definition, even when they are adopted arbitrarily in diverse contexts. Note how in this ecstatic prose, 'TV' and 'philosophy', etc. are seen as equivalent discursive domains, and how phenomenology inspires the emergentist awe of the writers.

The decade after Sokal has seen a proliferation of transcendent anti-science writing. It seems to offer an alternative to fields as diverse as psychology, geography, and sociology – all of which once unproblematically concerned actual people and their social and cultural lives. In the new discourses these fields are seen as vulgarly scientistic and illiberal because (to return to my starting point) they write about 'life' in terms of 'closed structures'; they ignore 'affect' and 'becomings'. 'Human sciences' are passé because they are naïvely objectivist. By contrast, those of us not schooled in Cultural Studies' appropriation of Theory might see them as sensibly empirical and sceptical. Moreover, they demand open-minded humility in the face of complex reality that refuses facile, purely verbal, pseudo-explanation of the kind I have considered in this chapter.

If any more examples of the infiltration of animistic metaphors into political/ethical and sociological writing are needed, let me cite another of my colleagues, this time rejecting what she calls 'categorical imperatives' [*sic*] in favour of, again, 'becoming'. Gay Hawkins invokes William Connolly's post-Deleuzian notion of a '*politics* of becoming' to analyse an ethics of waste and its relationships with people and public policy/governance. Again, 'affect' and 'becoming' effortlessly perform a lot of Theoretical work:

> Connolly's argument about responsiveness resonates with Deleuze and Guattari's idea of the body as a plane of affects: 'Affects are becomings ... [W]e know nothing about a body until we know what it can do, in other words, what its affects are, how they can enter into composition with other affects, with the affects of another body'. For Connolly, responsiveness is a condition of possibility, it opens up lines of mobility and difference within the self, and it is something that can be cultivated ... It involves work on the self in the interests of recognising the plurivocality of being and denaturalising identity as stasis or essence. (Hawkins 2006: 38)

I have no wish to analyse this verbal cascade in detail, merely to draw attention to its register of psychological-sounding processes. Note that the conclusion points us away from 'essence' or 'stasis', perhaps away from people as actual physical/psychological entities, towards pure abstraction and indeterminism. I am just as bemused as my grammar-check is by propositions such as 'affects are becomings ...', especially given Crandall's gloss on this concept that I quoted at length above. At the very least, I think Cultural Studies apprentices might expect 'affect' to be invoked with a greater degree of definitional consistency than it is in this example.

Theory writers perform complex metaphysical gymnastics to avoid a realist notion of the psychological subject (as we have seen in Chapter 3). They idealize pleasure and pain and avoid explanatory accounts of people's experiences and identities (including their sexual or other tastes) because they seem to allow no systematically theorized 'drives' or motivational systems (an issue central to Psychology since Freud at least). Individual histories of fear and flight – that is, responses mediated by known physiological mechanisms – do not seem to be what affect is about. But then, what does the term designate?

The obsessive avoidance of 'foundationalism' seems to imply that no 'basic' qualities of human nature can be postulated to provide narrative explanatory accounts of social or psychological phenomena: Marxist 'labour' is transcended, Freud's 'drives' are expunged, Darwin's natural selection processes are overlooked in favour of 'concepts with which to think' – to think, it seems, about no particular aspects of material processes or objects. 'Affect' would seem to offer Theory the opportunity to paper over these lacunae. But, on the evidence of the all-too-typical examples above, this seems unlikely. Postulating affect-drenched becomings presents no unique insight into culturally and psychologically intense experiences and activities. Immersing oneself (oops, one's subjectivity?) in an opera or identifying with a violent boxer may be culturally significant experiences, but interpreting them in terms of all-purpose 'affect' and references to Spinoza or Deleuze may show more about the commentator's knowledge of the Theorists' vocabularies than it does about the phenomena themselves.

Becoming Ontological – The Student's Problem

I have illustrated the 'process ontology' espoused by followers of Deleuze, in Chapters 1 and 2. Leaving aside the question of why students need to accept metaphysical novelties in order to study culture, semiotics, or identity, the literature that permeates much of Cultural Studies' curricula presents just such ideas as central to understanding an array of humanities perennials – 'memory', speech and 'speaking', and the psychological subject (discussed in detail in Chapter 3). Here is Elizabeth Grosz spelling out some of the interrelated tenets of 'transcendental empiricism' (*pace* Massumi and Deleuze, to whom I have already alluded). I ask the reader to peruse this passage carefully, with the assurance that I have quoted the text accurately:

> It is not as though there is a real world (realism) that is repeated virtually in the subject (as ideal). The actual is constant becoming virtual. The peculiar virtual of the human, however, is that it reverses the actual-virtual order of becoming. A body becomes virtual by organising itself into a subject ... this virtual effect then posits itself as the actual ground ... For Deleuze, then, the reactivism of the subject is overcome not by denying the subject – the death or critique of the subject – but by affirming the subject as a virtual effect, then by multiplying movements of subjective 'virtuality'. This is why transcendental empiricism is connected to a multiplication of voices, not as expressions of a subject but as expressions *per se*. The expression is, then, an assemblage. And if expression is understood from the concept of eternal return, it is not located within the self-recognising subject of time (a fold that turns back on itself) but distributed spatially, nomadically (an unfolding). (Grosz 1999: 131)

Even allowing for the terminology derived from Deleuze, and accepting that the passage concerns abstract postulates, the student of culture who tries to decipher this passage faces insurmountable difficulties: it continually equivocates about the subject and object of its sentences. Hence, a kind of magical thinking is evidenced in which bodies, subjects, effects, and the 'actual' seem have the logical status of personifications, each possessing its own agency (e.g., 'a body becomes virtual by organising itself'). Fundamentally, the student's concern must centre on the nature of the claims (if any) being made here: is the whole passage meant to be no more than definitional? If so, are the terms (such as 'expressions', 'body', 'effects', 'voices', 'time', etc.) intended to mean what they mean in everyday English? If not, is the sleight of hand here that the passage only 'works' if one comes to it *already accepting that they are being used prosaically*, even though the writing obscures this very understanding of the many everyday terms it willingly borrows?

If nothing else, the Grosz passage is a striking illustration of the educational dilemma faced by Cultural Studies novices when very general philosophically complex, but intricately interrelated concepts are assumed to be part of their vocabulary. The various terms she employs are all defined in terms of one another; they form a closed circle of postulates. Students have to accept the whole system, or remain estranged from the insights it purports to provide. It is as though Grosz has to use language like 'a switchman who locates a freight car by moving everything in the yard', to quote Norman Mailer's metaphor about Hubert Humphrey's laboured syntax (Rich 2008: 9).

Once a metaphysical system is entered, the whole creation has to be accepted by the reader. This is because the terms or concepts only make sense in relation to one another; they cannot be used in empirical propositions in the way that students of the humanities habitually assume. So, for example, one can understand how 'a body becomes virtual by organising itself into a subject' only if one also knows the particular (peculiar?) sense given to each of the three principal terms in the proposition. (And the reader surely needs one term, at least, to refer to something other than words, to designate real situations, objects, etc.).

Unsurprisingly, most students feel forced to respond only rhetorically to writing such as I have considered in relation to affect, by peppering their essays with words borrowed from Theory-speak. Worse, should the student also be reading academic psychology, anthropology or sociology, they will have no option but to compartmentalize in discrete boxes their separate disciplinary knowledge. They will learn to inoculate themselves against Theory that they hardly comprehend but which they fear might undermine their epistemological certainty about other fields of study.

Affect extraordinaire: Horse Sense?

Lisa Blackman's 2008 undergraduate textbook, *The Body: The Key Concepts*, invokes 'affect' to interpret the 'socially-constructed body'. She presents a theorization of socially-located 'bodies' as subjects, and sees the subject-in-general (as I called it in Chapters 3 and 4) as consisting of, or in, 'enactment' or 'performance'. Along the way she argues that 'sociologized' biology is the 'generative force of matter', thereby continuing Theory's metaphysical interpretation of mundane psycho-social and bio-social phenomena. Blackman argues that affect and related concepts help to avoid the mind-body problem – a metaphysical impediment that she attributes to Cartesian dualism. Instead of postulating interacting idealist 'substances' – in place of 'mind' magically affecting 'body' – contemporary body theorists describe psychological processes as social events, often mediated by 'affect'. I want to consider briefly Blackman's adoption of this term, and to argue that it is used in a circular or vacuous way when proposed as an alternative to psychologically realist (deterministic, non-teleological and non-idealist) accounts of the phenomena she chooses to consider as exemplars of the conceptual virtues of 'Body Theory'. Again I draw attention to the way in which theorists of cultural and social relationships between and amongst people (and between people and other animal species in Blackman's case) offer elaborately abstract re-interpretations of prosaic phenomena such as animals performing circus tricks, and writes at length about other putative relationships between humans and their pets. Surprisingly, despite her empirical-sounding descriptions of such relationships, the Theorist ignores potentially contradictory evidence such as counter-examples that might encourage a more realist and less grandiose analysis.

Blackman explicitly rejects Psychology in favour of 'Body Theory' by discussing what all Anglo-American students of academic psychology will recognize as an old pedagogical chestnut – the case of the horse that seemed to be able to do mental arithmetic. Psychology students know him as 'Clever Hans'. Blackman explains:

> Hans appeared to be able to solve fairly complex multiplication puzzles by stamping his hooves. In 1904 a commission of people led by Carl Stumpf, who was the director of the Berlin Psychological Institution, was assembled to judge and evaluate (these) claims. The members concluded that either Hans was possessed of exceptional intelligence and/or had psychic abilities ... Hans became a test case in experimental psychology for the problem of social influence. (Blackman 2008: 39)

Psychologists later showed that in fact Hans was responding to small cues given by his handler, such as raising his head when the answer to an arithmetical puzzle had been 'counted' out and thus 'represented' by the horse's hoof stamps. No magical powers were required of Clever Hans, or, for that matter, of his owner. However, Blackman prefers a more complex 'explanation' for the events that seemed to show Hans to have been a horse of unusual sense. She emphasizes the 'relationality' between the horse and the trainer, and the possibility of 'attunement' between them. She cites, with approval, Despret (2004), who 'argues that the case of Hans makes visible the capacity of human and horse to transform each other to such a degree that they are affected by and affect each other' (Blackman 2008: 21). This is an oddly complicated way of describing simple phenomena. Of course, animals and humans interact (in Hans's case, per medium of appropriately-timed lumps of sugar). Similarly, when equestrian contestants in Olympic events train and form an ensemble or team with their equine charges, the duos are capable of complex, repeatable performances.

In such cases, horses' qualities (such as the ability to learn complex behaviours), and the reward regimes that their trainers implement to teach them, are usually thought of as the explanation of the phenomena in question. The trainer/riders might feel 'at one' with their four-footed partners, but so might a pilot with their aircraft or a surgeon with the organ on which they are operating. No novel psycho-sociological meta-concepts seem to be needed to make sense of these situations. Nor do Theory's versions of them lead to any new insights, despite the enthusiastic claims of their proponents.

Blackman goes on to argue that the conception of 'the body' in experimental psychology (and in folk psychology, I would add) is mechanistic (my term) and fails to take into account the role of 'affect' and the 'becoming' that constitute the social life of bodies (both animal and human, it would seem, from her example). She speaks of new realities coming into being through such relationships. Of course, this is true in the sense that every performance of a behavioural sequence is unique in certain respects, but that insight would not seem to herald an ontological revolution. I cannot reproduce all her analyses, but her crucial point is that bodies are 'performed' interactively, so to speak, and thus there can be no 'clear distinction between the individual and the social, the biological and the cultural and the self and other' (Blackman 2008: 45). This leads her to a discussion of 'emotional contagion' and then to consideration of Freudian 'projection' and other 'relational' psychological phenomena. She emphasizes 'becoming' rather than 'singular' and 'separate' bodies: 'That is the mixing and interconnection between self and other [that] does not reveal an authentic separate realm but rather the capacity we all have for being affected and affecting the other' (2008: 44).

A less metaphysically-inclined psychologist might object that this 'affect-becoming' paradigm prevents precise analysis of many phenomena that *do* involve actual bodies. It fails to allow that bodies have any real qualities – for example, that horses and humans *in fact* can only enter into particular kinds of relationships and that these depend in part on their distinguishable and distinct 'bodies'. They are distinct species, after all. Secondly, Blackman seems to misunderstand deterministic psychology, thinking that it rules out in advance any attempt to conceptualize social influence and encounters, not to mention social ensembles and the changing 'performances' of affective relationships. But, on the contrary, Psychology since Clever Hans's time (or thereabouts) has been almost exclusively concerned with the ways by which biological and cultural phenomena are mutually determining. To analyse such relationships coherently means that *conceptually separable entities* need to be distinguished if they are to be *empirically isolated* and their *respective causal roles inferred*. In short, Blackman tries to describe a knowable, dynamic social world but is reluctant to resort to any descriptive predicates that could refer to the qualities of particular species, particular situations or to relevant mechanisms of putative causation of anything in particular. Therefore no methodological advantage is demonstrated as a result of her reconceptualised socio-psychology.

As with the 'post-human' speculations discussed in Chapter 5, 'body theorists' seem to have thrown away the very postulates that would have allowed them to understand actual, particular social-psychological situations and the ways by which bodies are implicated in these. They have then multiplied concepts rather hopefully to explain, or to describe at least, aspects of complex interactions (such as training one's horse), although these sound like no more than romantic attempts to transcend what the writers see as the mechanistic assumptions of academic psychology.

Many of the newly-minted concepts of Body Theory are so vague that they offer no explanatory information about the phenomena being analysed. Moreover, the writers simply ignore any situations that might pose difficulties for the meta-theoretical assumptions of their accounts. This can be seen by asking the kind of question that psychologists routinely ask of their own explanations: Are there any counter-examples that might show one's analyses to be circular or 'purely verbal'? For instance, Blackman calls certain equine-human relationships 'attunement', and sees them as examples of mutual 'becoming'. But are less socially-pleasant relationships also examples of this concept? Are 'attunement' and 'becoming' equally useful ways of understanding a Nazi dog-trainer's relationship with his Alsatian charge? And what of the family pet, harmoniously attuned to the routines of its owners, which nevertheless attacks and savages a child of the household? It is no help to say, *after the event*, that these cases were not 'really' cases of attunement or affective relationships, otherwise the attacks would not have occurred. That would beg the question. A 'theory' of social relationships such as pet-human ensembles needs to account for the *variety* of these relationships and *their limits*, such as when 'affect' turns into hostility, if it is to provide a contestable explanation of what actually happens in particular classes of social situations. And, as Body Theory tries to rewrite Sociology, understanding distinguishable types of social situations would seem to be a pre-requisite for its methodological success.

Body Theory purports to be realist and to understand biology as always 'subject to change'. Biology is 'socialized', or 'enacted'; the nature of Nature is always mediated (Blackman 2008: 130). Of course, this is true in an important sense. However, this general point does not mean that one can never understand *aspects* of biological processes independently of their social mediation. For example, body scarring *can be described for particular explanatory purposes* independently of the social meaning and identity membership that may be expressed through body scarification. Theory seems to have misunderstood this methodological point, without which sciences would not be able to make any claims about reality. Knowledge claims such as those of biology and of psychology are *aspectual*, and *contexutalized*. They need not be interpreted as universal or metaphysical. Each particular proposition respectively *predicates particular aspects of particular classes of phenomena*, within particular theoretical contexts. This allows scientists to make empirical proposals about the states of things in the world, so to speak, but only in relation to the aspects they nominate. Psychologists are not committed to mind-body dualism when they describe Hans's performance of 'mental arithmetic'; nor do they necessarily endorse the view that biological phenomena are fixed and invariable or immune to ecological influence when they study species qua species.

Relations such as those that held between Clever Hans and his owner during the first decade of the twentieth century were several and can be spoken about separately. They do not imply a new methodological set of assumptions about biological 'relationality' per se. Theory analysts often write as though terms with metaphysical provenance (like 'becoming' and 'affect') are, after all, only descriptive empirical terms when used to discuss mundane social or biological reality. This practice is as methodologically careless as it is educationally pernicious.

Equally worrying for someone aiming to teach students how to think about social and psychological phenomena is the facile way in which relationships between a horse and a person can be analysed without referring to anything in particular about horses as a species (e.g., their sensory capacities and ability to learn responses through reward regimes), let alone about the participants' histories of learning from each other. Clever Hans's mathematical accomplishments were not achieved without at least a few well-timed sugar lumps. It is all very well to describe the 'relationality' of such affecting phenomena, but it is *particular* relations that count (if you will excuse the pun). Of course, one can also describe such joint behaviours as 'performances', but is there any epistemological or educational advantage in doing so?

Chapter 7

Real Experience, Un-Real Science

Pooh began to feel a little more comfortable, because when you are a Bear of Very Little Brain, and you Think of Things, you find sometimes that a Thing which seemed very Thingish inside you is quite different when it gets out into the open and has other people looking at it.
AA Milne

To imagine you need an external social situation and physical stuffs.
Crispin Sartwell

This chapter examines the curious Cultural Studies attempt to rewrite biological and psychological 'science as Theory'. I consider further Lisa Blackman's textbook on 'the body' understood from a New Humanities perspective, and then examine Brian Massumi's boast to break the ontological shackles of biological psychology by borrowing and coining terms to refer to 'infra-empirical' processes in the pulsating psychophysical worlds that he thinks academic psychology overlooks. Both authors emphasize 'relationality' – that is, relations between living things and their social and physical environments, and the 'new realities' that can be postulated when the world is understood as 'process' rather than as 'dumb matter' and 'substance'. Their eclectic approaches, although very different in many respects, might be called 'phenomenological/ecological' to draw attention to the writers' wholesale criticism of scientific understandings of 'processes that operate on multiple registers of sensation', beyond 'standard rhetorical and semiotic models'.

Blackman writes not about what 'the body' *is*, but about what bodies do and what they can become through various kinds of *performance*. This enables her to 'radically refigure the idea of the body as *substance* or *entity* and even as distinctly *human*' (Blackman 2008: 1), ideas that I have considered in previous chapters. Recall that 'essentialism' is a principal issue with which Cultural Studies methodology is concerned (see Chapter 3). Here I want to focus on the methodological consequences of Blackman's transcendental sociology insofar as it proclaims a revolution, in regard to biological causality especially.

Massumi takes a different tack to transcending the psychologically mundane. He labels his approach 'materialist' and 'hyper-realist'. However, I will argue that he interprets as referring to psychologically real phenomena, various abstract nouns that sound suspiciously like crude reifications (such as 'variation', 'force' and 'potential'). To 'snatch experience from the jaws of science', he resorts to phenomenological description, hoping it will allow him to depict 'infra-empirical' realities. Whereas Blackman is little concerned with what goes on 'inside the organism', Massumi is happy to write at both the molecular-physiological and macro-social levels with a confidence that might alarm a neurophysiologist or endocrinologist. As humanities writers, both Blackman and Massumi allow themselves the luxury of hedging their bets about determinism. This is central to their respective sleights of hand. I will argue that it allows them to avoid the responsibility of making testable predictions about anything in particular, the very stuff of the sciences they so grandly rewrite. So, where Theory is concerned, readers are implicitly invited to 'take it or leave it'. However, I will try to confront these writers' accounts of psychological reality with methodological criteria that they so eloquently evade. Each writer dismisses the methods of 'science', and misunderstands the caution and circumspection with which biological and psychological knowledge claims are usually justified in the academic disciplines they disparage.

Although it overlaps with some of the concerns of earlier analyses, this chapter could be read in isolation by anyone interested in what Theory means when it transcends the mundane practices of conventional sociology, psychology and biology. It may help the reader, however, to think of this chapter as an extension of my discussion of 'the subject', 'post-humanism' and 'affect'.

Moving Science: The Body in Theory

'*Is there anything natural about the human body? Is this still a viable concept for organising, examining and reflecting upon the body as an object of study within the humanities?*' So begins Blackman's recent textbook summarizing ideas about the intersections of what were once the disciplines of Biology, Sociology, Psychology and Philosophy. She promises to 'radically refigure the idea of the body as substance or entity and even as distinctly human' (Blackman 2008: 1). Because it is so eclectic and ambitious, so clearly a capital-T Theory textbook (in the sense I have discussed in previous chapters), *The Body* throws into sharp relief many of the educational issues that flow from recent post-disciplinary scholarship, especially as these relate to rewriting perennial psychobiological and biosocial questions.

Methodologically, Blackman's textbook mixes phenomenological with empirical description, ignoring the ontological consequences of this conflation (a practice I have illustrated in many ways throughout this book). She invokes scientific evidence about what she calls 'vitality', and 'liveness', and postulates 'affect' and 'enactment' as both cause and effect in relation to 'the feeling body'. However, the evidence cited is recontextualized into a 'process ontology' (including, predictably, 'becomings' that know no 'be-goings') and into social constructivist epistemology. This purports to form the basis for Blackman's challenge to Cartesian (body/mind) dualism, the metaphysical error that infects all psychological science, it seems.

As the phrase '*the* body' implies, her approach takes as its own theoretical object what one might call 'bodies-in-general' in order to interpret their different relations with cultural and technological factors. In this, she is 'culturalist', to again use Terry Eagleton's phrase, although Blackman is happy to discuss what other disciplines might call 'diseases' or 'abnormalities' of the body that sound to be anything but socially constructed per se. Her introductory précis promises that the book will 'connect ... up some of the gaps and anomalies encountered [in the cross-disciplinary field] and attempt ... to further inject aliveness and vitality into a body that for many years has only been an absent present in social and cultural theory' (Blackman 2008: 13). My argument is that this injection proves to be less than therapeutically efficacious, despite Blackman's ambition to rectify the maladies of sciences that see the body as 'substance' and her desire to 'trouble ... the idea that the biological and cultural are two separate, two absolutely discrete entities that somehow interact [sic]' (2008: 81).

To help students to think about bodies relieved of the burden of substances, five chapters overview topics such as:

The socially constructed body
Agency and the body
Embodiment
Becoming (horse-human)
Emotional contagion
Affective transmission
Bodily markers of respectability
Touch
Taste
The mouth
Healthism and the body
The body multiple
Modulation
Corporeal thinking

As it is an undergraduate textbook, *The Body* concludes with a long list of 'questions for essays and classroom discussion'. These are nothing if not challenging, and many ask that students understand and criticize epistemological and ontological positions central to Western Philosophy, and/or reinterpret in Body Theory terms, the scientific knowledge and basic concepts of modern Psychology, Psychiatry and Sociology. The questions seem to imply one or a few correct answers, answers found in the various chapters of the book itself. They include:

Discuss the difference between approaching the body as a substance or entity, and the approaches which focus on 'the body' as a process.

What is meant by the concept of dualism?

What does it mean to study bodies as 'unfinished entities'? (cf. Question 1, above).

How does Despret's ... conception of becoming transform how we might understand non-verbal communication?

To what extent can class be considered a form of corporeal capital?

Discuss some of the different ways in which the concept of 'bodily affectivity' has been used to understand the enactment of difference, and what does this introduce into the study of bodily dispositions?

Why is history important for understanding sense organization?

How does the study of biomediation challenge the historical separation between the humanities and the life and biological sciences?

At the very least, this mode of assessing students' understanding of a textbook is likely to encourage predictably glib 'Theory' essays that ignore the respective epistemological and methodological contexts of the disciplinary knowledge they are expected to cite: for example, 'class' (Marx?), 'dualism' (Descartes, and more recent mental philosophy), 'affect' (Freud, and many other psychologists), 'bodily dispositions' (dispositional concepts have a long history in academic psychology and are difficult to analyse coherently). Incidentally, Blackman's book also canvasses the distinction between 'subjects' and 'subject positions', considered in Chapter 4 above.

Apart from assuming that students have an advanced understanding of Western metaphysics, perhaps the most troubling educational consequences of these demanding questions are that they meld, quite arbitrarily, various methodological paradigms, and encourage students to do likewise. At the same time readers are invited, on the basis of a few historical examples that illustrate naïve biologism, to dismiss all realist psychological knowledge as passé. Blackman instances several examples of essentialism and reductionism – biological-psychological chestnuts that cry out for methodological critique (these include eugenics, naïve social Darwinism, and vulgar biochemical explanations of psychological 'states'). For instance, *The Body* highlights as an egregious instance of such scientism, Emile Kraepelin's characterization of *dementia praecox*, dating from 1919 (Blackman 2008: 18–19).

Kraepelin's crudely essentialist nomenclature is an example on which many Psychology students still cut their own critical teeth, but it is certainly not typical of current psychiatric science. Indeed, the history of how *dementia praecox* has been reconceptualized as 'schizophrenia', and that label itself vigorously debated, shows how psychologists have self-critically come to understand psychiatric conditions as 'relational' and not as mere 'substances' or discrete pathogens that cause 'symptoms'. This and Blackman's other examples seem like proverbial 'straw men' against which to mount a critique of biologism in Psychology, as few if any psychologists would disagree with her position.

Blackman argues that some (all?) common medical conditions cannot be adequately described in physiological terms, presumably because this would be essentialist (recall that essentialism involves attributing fixed physical attributes to a phenomenon, such as when 'gender' is equated with hormonal/physiological qualities). Instead, cultural descriptors must be invoked to capture the 'processual' and relational aspects of what common scientific sense mistakenly label as conditions *of* bodies. This re-theorization allows the lived experiences of people to be thought of as 'practices' per se, and this, presumably, means that, say, the disease entities implied in medical nomenclature should be jettisoned in favour of non-reductive dynamic understandings. As will be seen, however, it remains unclear just what ontological status is claimed for the conventionally-designated physiological conditions that Body

Theory re-describes. Blackman does allow that, in her approach to corporeal or materiality, 'bodies are real but they are also made, remade and even unmade. They are literally brought into being [sic] through practices and modes of enactment' (2008: 123–4). However, this is paradoxical at best, and begs the question of what makes pathological conditions pathological in the first place because pathogens seem to be understood also as what she calls 'practices'. What she probably means is that 'what bodies mean socially', so to speak, is continually renegotiated – a very different proposition. However, her discussion of a medical condition, its effects and its social manifestation, makes it difficult to be certain that this is, in fact, her position.

Avoiding essentialism and biological reductionism, Blackman illustrates why we need to think of 'the multiple body' as multiple 'performances' by discussing the unlikely case of how bodies '*do hypoglycaemia*' (her phrase). Describing the performance of hypoglycaemic symptoms as 'interactions' and 'incorporations of bits and pieces of the world around it', Blackman is able to conclude that because each hypoglycaemic event is different from others, 'what we witness is a multiplicity, rather than a fixity and the assumption of one static underlying object: hypoglycaemia' (2008: 124). So, on her analysis, a person's low blood sugar is not usefully thought of as a discrete cause of some identifiable, certainly no 'fixed', class of symptomatic phenomena. What medicine calls 'symptoms' come into being (only?) through performance, as it were.

One might ask why this circuitous way of denying the role of pathogens and particular malfunctioning physiologies is necessary for theoretical correctness. One might also ask whether it is coherent. Surely all the class of 'performances' involving hypoglycaemia do have something in common, otherwise Blackman could not coherently identify the events that she is analysing for their similarities to, and differences from, other such 'performances'. That is to say, her way of putting the observation begs the question of whether there is a common (causal) factor in all such 'events', the very point of biological explanation (as opposed to cultural analysis). Indeed, this is the very reason that biological accounts claim to be causal – they are essentialist to the extent that they hypothesize specific conditions as *necessary or sufficient* for other kinds or classes of events to occur.

Acknowledging that each hypoglycaemic 'event' or 'performance' is unique tells us nothing about the functions of sugar as a component of human blood, or about the effects on particular classes of organisms that follow from changes in its 'level'. Moreover, it might be added, Blackman's circuitous rhetoric for avoiding causal biological factors could be profoundly offensive to people whose individual 'hypoglycaemic events' (what we might once have called their 'symptomatology') are involuntary, disempowering, and incapacitating. We might ask Blackman whether life-threatening diabetic comas should also be thought of as cultural performances, as unique 'doings'? 'Performances' and 'doings' sound optional or voluntary. Dying during a diabetic coma certainly is not! (Perhaps we should we put 'dying' in scare quotes to allow us to think about it less naïvely, that is, more 'culturally').

If Body Theory is not to be committed to a naïve kind of selective determinism (some events being arbitrarily exempt from the question of their cause), it needs to show that biology is *necessarily reductionist* or *essentialist in relevant respects* to the cases it champions as exemplary 'performances'. Blackman does not do this. Instead her confusion only deepens when she asks her readers to think about 'selective serotonin re-uptake inhibitors' (SSRIs). Do these 'challenge the view of personhood' organized around the 'fiction of autonomous selfhood', as she asserts? Does neuropharmacology show that '... rather than becoming-other [*sic*] ... we are potentially becoming more biological' (2008: 115)? This is an ironic choice of example, because one might have thought that if anyone were aware that the mind and the body are not separate 'substances' and that selfhood is not 'autonomous', it would be deterministic psychologists and those students who have found themselves (or what they think of as themselves) caught up in 'performances' of 'depression'. Indeed, those who think they *suffer from* rather than *perform* depression are likely to believe in a rather crude brand of biological determinism about this painful and debilitating condition that is anything but voluntary, however apparently unique 'its' many performances. It is possible to see in these examples how Theorists' equivocation about determinism leads to ethically and politically questionable consequences – ironically, consequences they seem to have struggled to avoid.

Cultural Studies' attempt to disown conventional cause-effect science may lead to risible consequences. These may result from the incoherent attempt 'to say everything at once' about a complex relational phenomenon. Coherent discourse is propositional, and speakers nominate discrete grammatical subjects of which specific predications can be made. For this reason, all verbal descriptions of events draw attention to *certain aspects* of the phenomena in question, and not to other aspects. How could we communicate about any complex situation other than 'aspectually'? Cultural Studies predictably focuses on the *cultural and socially relational* aspects of phenomena to which biological factors may only infrequently be causally relevant. But it is unclear why this should imply a theoretical revolution, the rejection of all biological science, and incidentally liberate students from the shackles of Cartesian dualism.

As I have argued, a major philosophical issue remains unresolved in 'Body Theory'. It is unclear whether its proponents are committed to the assumption of determinism. Although Blackman's pejorative reference to the 'fiction of autonomous selfhood' implies that it is, she also considers 'agency and the body' in rather ambivalent terms. She tries to avoid what might be just a new form of determinist (albeit *socially* determinist) analysis by somewhat hopefully postulating 'aliveness or vitality' as irreducible aspects of bodies. This is intended to prevent 'the body' from being reduced to physiological processes, but also to save it from complete social determinism. And, as I have mentioned, her book generally invokes 'relationality' and 'affect' to fill out a theoretical account of bodies existing only in performances.

It is not necessarily a criticism of academic Biology or Psychology to write sociologically or 'relationally' about physiological factors such as blood sugar levels. Of course bodies feel and behave in particular ways under the influence of chemical changes, and each symptomatic event is unique. But showing that unique events share certain etiological or phenomenological characteristics is a first step towards trying to understand them empirically. That is where science begins – classifying and naming, looking for regularities in the putative causal factors involved in identifiable *classes of events*. Science is not *necessarily* 'reductionist' or 'essentialist' when it makes claims about biological causes and conditions. Nor, *pace* Blackman, is it necessary to 'multiply realities' in order to explore relationships between bodies and artefacts, people and cultures, subjects and history. Educationally, such metaphysically eccentric postulates are likely, at best, to confuse students unless they are justified in philosophical detail.

I accept that Cultural Studies is concerned with the 'meaning' of the body in cultural relationships (e.g., as signifying gender, or embodying 'disability') and not with the nature and causes of bodies' qualities in an empirical sense. However, to study the former one must assume *that bodies are of certain kinds*, and that means that they are carriers of certain qualities or characteristics and are, or can be, implicated only in *particular kinds of causal relationships, and not in others*. That is, bodies are not infinitely plastic; they cannot simply be 'talked into existence'. They can be involved only in particular kinds of actual material, semiotic and social relationships. Blackman tacitly acknowledges this by restricting the various 'bodies' of her analyses to a small class. But it is a rather arbitrary list. Worse, it is potentially infinite: she could just as easily have postulated other 'bodies' such as 'the athletic body', 'the mortal body', 'the copulatory body', 'the mechanical body', etc. Indeed, it is these aspects of bodies on which anatomy, gerontology, endocrinology and fitness training respectively concentrate and, of course, these sub-disciplines allow that the contexts within which people's bodies work and change are relevant to understanding them. The crucial question in each body-as-performance case is whether an exclusively culturalist analysis offers new knowledge of some aspects of human behaviour or human 'nature' (there I have said it): does it enable new ways of formulating propositions about some actual situations, events, entities or states of affairs? Body Theory, as a sub-field of Cultural Studies, needs to do more than simply rewrite Biology and Psychology in novel vocabularies if it is to present contestable ways of understanding particular aspects of human (or even 'post-human') subjectivity, behaviour and experience.

Vital Phenomenology

'Phenomenology' refers to the careful description of the phenomena of experience, undertaken free of any epistemological preconceptions (Bullock & Trombley 2000: 645–6). A non-psychologist might see this as an obvious source of knowledge about how people feel and think. It is no surprise that Theorists whom I have discussed throughout this book mix analyses of experience with their more objective claims about psychological phenomena. Indeed, the examples of ostensibly psychological theorizing flowing from Deleuze that I see epitomized in Massumi clearly owe a debt to the turn of the twentieth-century phenomenological philosopher, Henri Bergson. This is not to say that Cultural Studies in general is wedded to phenomenology, or that its proponents explicitly develop an alternative to mainstream Psychology. However, they do generally see Psychology as narrowly empirical, and often dismiss it as 'positivistic', by which they mean that it accumulates isolated 'facts' believed to be value-free and universally true. This may be a caricature of Psychology, but Cultural Studies has reacted against just this parody, especially when it finds inspiration in older schools of psychological enquiry such as Bergsonian phenomenology.

To understand the context from which Cultural Studies neo-psychology emerges, let me briefly list a few key ideas in Bergson's influential approach to psychological philosophy. He postulates:

- A 'creative', process-based notion of evolution and of life ('shells bursting into fragments, each itself a shell' is a Bergsonian image)
- Phenomenological analyses of temporality and of memory itself (e.g. as analogous to experiences of cinema)
- Teleological emergentism (that is, purpose-directed analyses of phenomena that 'emerge' in unpredictable ways from other phenomena)
- Anti-rationalism and the celebration of 'intuition'
- 'Becoming' and change, seen as the province of 'intuition' rather than 'reason'

It is not important to fully understand Bergson in order to appreciate Cultural Studies' attraction to phenomenology. However, many ideas that echo throughout recent post-structuralist Cultural Studies clearly derive from phenomenology of his kind. They provide a theoretical vocabulary with which to replace most of what Anglophone Psychology and Philosophy have taken for granted during the post-war period. Notwithstanding the many objections to Bergson (neatly summarized as early as 1946 by Bertrand Russell), the antagonism of more recent Theory to empirical social sciences, even to the biological and physical sciences, has been fuelled by the rejection of reason and scientific method, and hence by scepticism about the very possibility of 'objective knowledge'. So let me return to the celebrated example of these tendencies which I introduced in Chapters 1 and 2, and which were all published *after* the Sokal furore had subsided.

As I noted in earlier chapters, the psychological (yet putatively anti-empirical) assumptions of Deleuze's 'post-structuralism' have been taken up by many Cultural Studies writers, especially those who wish to move away from 'humanism', 'reductionism', and other alleged sins of post-Enlightenment science. Digital media and 'virtual reality' have led Deleuze's translator, Massumi (2002), to adopt the kinds of concepts I have tried to explicate earlier, to describe cultural and corporeal reality. To introduce the aims of his book, *Parables for the Virtual*, I quote below its dust-jacket summary, which outlines more clearly than does the author the ambition of the essays it contains. The publisher, Duke University Press, advertises the work as relevant to 'Philosophy/Cultural Studies/Science Studies'. The 'Science' in question includes Psychology, presumably, although the book takes issue with many conventional theories and meta-theories of the physical sciences as well. The cover notes read:

> In *Parables For The Virtual* Brian Massumi views the body and media such as television, film, and the internet as processes that operate on multiple registers of sensation beyond the reach of the reading techniques founded on the standard rhetorical and semiotic models. Renewing and assessing William James's radical empiricism and Henri Bergson's philosophy of perception through the filter of the postwar French philosophy of Deleuze, Guattari, and Foucault, Massumi links a cultural logic of variation to questions of movement, affect, and sensation. If such concepts are as fundamental as signs and significations, he argues, then a new set of theoretical issues appear, and with them potential new paths for the wedding of scientific and cultural theory. (Back cover text for Massumi 2002)

According to his supporters, Massumi aims to move beyond semiotic (and thus 'culturalist') accounts of psychosocial phenomena, yet to talk about experience in realist ways. Commendably, in my view, he is interested in what happens when people experience cultural, aesthetic, and, indeed, any sensory or perceptual phenomena. He therefore confronts his readers with his cultural/aesthetic analyses based on extreme phenomenology. However, as I will show, this is soon mixed with his own brand of reified mentalism and an ecstatic vitalism. Remember that Deleuze has written on Bergson and Spinoza. Massumi alludes to these and also to many twentieth-century psychologists and philosophers to sustain his ontological speculations. However, these become well-nigh incoherent, especially when he tries to analyse what have been long-regarded as psychological questions concerning *perception/sensation*, *memory* and *thought* processes, and when he criticizes, among other things, representationalist models of *language*. His world is imbued with 'virtualities', 'potentials', 'becomings', and 'infra-empirical' forces that are supposed to render scientific Psychology passé. Not only does 'affect' animate 'life' (in general), but 'the virtual' (a kind of infinite potential actualization or latency) inheres in nature's (or should that be culture's?) ever-changing processes.

In the fairly typical passage that I quote at length below, Massumi piles words upon words to exhibit a kind of frenzied vitalism. The reader will note how many psychological processes (such as 'anticipation') are given no grammatical or actual (psychological) subject. Along with other relational terms, such as 'connectability', and various processes and states including 'potential' and 'latency', they work as purely verbal abstractions although they sound like realist referring terms:

> Every creature connecting with a flower will think-perceive it differently, extending the necessity of its perception into the only-thought of possibility to a varying degree ... The flower is each of the thought-perceptions in which it is implicated, to whatever degree of thought-perception. Which is not to say that there are as many flowers as there are

florally-conjoined creatures. The flower-thing is *all* of the thought-perceptions in which it is implicated. Latent in the flower are all of the differential conjunctions it may enter into. The flower as a thing 'in itself', is its connectability with other things outside itself. That connectability is not of the order of action or thought-out anticipation and is therefore not in the mode of possibility. It is the order of *force*. Each connection is a shared plug-in to a force emitted or transmitted by the flower-thing. Like a light wave. The latency in this case is in the mode not of the possible but of energetic *potential*. There is more potentially emitted or transmitted by the flower than any necessary perception of it picks up on (more…). The bee's hungry or horny perception is not 'relative' to the flower. It is selective of it (*and* less). (Massumi 2002: 92)

As Massumi celebrates the phenomenological life of bees, this passage reminds one of Bergson's preference for instinct over intellect. Russell joked:

The division between intellect and instinct is fundamental in (Bergson's) philosophy … but in the main, intellect is the misfortune of man while instinct is seen at its best in ants, bees, and Bergson (1961: 358)

Whether they bring to the passage such contextual knowledge, readers might still be alienated by this way of 'protesting against naïve objectivism' (to quote another academic luminary, Isabell Stengers, praising Massumi). They may feel obliged to reach for Occam's razor (or Occam's harvester, perhaps, in this case). They are unlikely to know what to make of the all-purpose 'force' that animates the flower's connections to its world. In this they would be in good company, because such postulates sound entirely gratuitous. As I have already mentioned in another context, the philosopher Daniel Dennett concludes his recent book on 'obstacles to a science of consciousness' by dismissing Massumi-style forces as vitalist. He restates the standard critique of vitalism found in analytic philosophy and in scientific psychology which is that it postulates entities for which no empirical warrant is available: 'Vitalism – the insistence that there is some big mysterious extra ingredient in all living things – turns out to have been not a deep insight but a failure of imagination' (Dennett 2005: 178).

In a more detailed discussion (Bell 2003), I argued that Massumi's post-Deleuzian analysis epitomizes the tortuous philosophical problems that beset the recourse of Cultural Studies to phenomenology and to what Deleuze terms 'transcendental empiricism'. One example of this is Massumi's re-analysis of a classic psychology text-book example, the experimentally-produced effects reported by Katz (1935). Briefly, Katz showed that people misremembered the colour of personally-significant objects (their friends' eyes, for example). The revisionary analysis that Massumi provides to 'explain' this kind of phenomenon includes the following passage.

If, in the interval between triggering and testing by 'blue', the subject is not doing what the experimenter is doing – setting up a correspondence between a past and present perception – what exactly is he or she doing with color? Or is that even the right question? Isn't the question rather: What is color doing to the subject? For the subject is not even aware of the excess she is producing until the experimenter reports the results. Until then she is left in the belief that she has made the match. The exaggeration that she effectively produces is the result of some 'absolutely striking' peculiarity of color. The subject has been singularly struck by color. Color has struck, and without either the subject or the experimenter willing it so, it has exceeded. It has gone over the instituted line … as unwilled as it is unmatched by its human hosts. (Massumi 2002: 211)

Without belabouring the point, this way of speaking about the phenomenon of mismatching colours is clearly vitalist. Yet Massumi uses this to postulate the 'self-activity' of experience: 'When a color is interrogated by language it displays a self-insistent dynamic that commands itself to the instituted context, into which it breaks and enters, delivering itself to the questioning' [sic] (2002: 211).

The processes and the agents that this purports to describe are simply magical. They are no more than verbal pseudo-explanations, in no way alternative to the realist postulates of psychology. Note, for instance, how colour which is 'striking' becomes an agent or *thing that strikes*! And what are these 'self-insistent dynamics that command'? Why is 'excess' of colour a thing itself in his circular analysis? Surely, 'excess' of colour refers to the judgement made by the subject in the experimental situation; it is not an entity that can be extracted from this process.

The passages above are not alternatives to psychological analysis, not even 'hyperempiricist' psychology or useful phenomenology. They are circular, vitalist and therefore vacuous, because they postulate active causal agents with no other warrant than that Massumi can use any noun in a more or less grammatically-correct way. By so doing, he populates people's judgements and perceptions with a limitless cast of forces and causes, all sounding active and all working to produce the effect that the psychologist himself is accused of naïvely misunderstanding. If only Katz had discovered the 'excesses' and the striking peculiarity of colour. If only he hadn't missed the 'self-delivery or ingressive activity of experience', so that he could have understood that 'the excess of color slips into language between the experimenter and the subject' (Massumi 2002: 211).

If nothing else, this example highlights the incoherence that seems inevitably to arise when both 'reality' and 'perception' are analysed in subjective, idealist ways. In this regard, it is like the phenomenology of the bee's relation to the flower as a 'thought-perception' (above). But I should add that in Massumi's case this is ostensibly done in the interests of what he claims are a dynamic, 'radically empiricist', ontology and epistemology (not that he uses these conventional terms with any consistency). Massumi also calls the psychological theorizing he presents '*incorporeally materialistic, super (or hyper or radical) empiricism*'.

As my examples attest, it is not just an epistemological revolution that Massumi advocates – it is ontological. He proposes novel things in the world – things like 'excesses' and 'forces' – that are not equivalent to the specific kinds of forces that physical biology would postulate to analyse the phenomena he discusses. On the contrary, Cultural Studies has discovered more than the world of science can claim to understand, and it has found these wonderful things right under science's nose! This ignores the blatant problem with his own approach – that it makes no predictions about any actual psychological phenomena, and is entirely post hoc. Therefore it can never be genuinely explanatory: Massumi merely *redescribes the inexplicable in terms of the unknowable.*

Masumi proposes his Bergson-cum-Deleuze approach in the interests, he maintains, of developing a *materialist* account of culture, bringing the body and its 'sensings as significations' back 'into the picture' (2002: 4). Indeed, as the phrase 'sensings as significations' suggests, he thinks of his theorizing as a kind of semiotics, but he wants to 'part company with the most widespread concepts of coding (almost always Saussurian in inspiration)' (2002: 4). It is a curious paradox, to say the least, that he uses phenomenology to grasp what he calls, 'the real *in*corporeality of the concrete'. And he asserts that 'interfering affect' is 'independent of all physical dimensions' (which sounds as though it floats free of material reality). Not that many students of Cultural Studies would see this as problematic, of course. Few are schooled in the history of philosophy or psychology sufficiently to allow them to expect writers to demonstrate the advantages that flow from their particular methods of analysis relative to other approaches.

Neo- or *Non*-Psychology?

My instances of Theorizing are not ostensibly concerned with what usually marches under the banner of 'Psychology', yet 'sensings', 'sensations' and 'affects', not to mention 'perception', 'cognition', and ad hoc experiential concepts, inform much of Cultural Studies Theory. Massumi's unconventional versions of these concepts constitute his claim to revolutionary methodological significance. Indeed, his book has been hailed as one that 'transports us from the dicey intersection of movement and sensation, through insightful exploration of affect and body image, to a creative reconfiguration of the 'nature-culture continuum' (Connolly quoted in Massumi 2002, cover notes).

Massumi writes of his epistemology: 'If incorporeal materialism is an empiricism, it is a radical one, summed up by the formula: the *felt reality of a relation*' (2002: 16, emphasis in original). The 'virtual' of his title, *Parables for the Virtual: Movement, Affect, Sensation*, derives from the thesis of the essays, if one can discern a single dominant thesis, namely that '[t]he "real but abstract" incorporeality of the body is the virtual' (2002: 21). The final chapter, for instance, returns to this assertion, reopening the question of what 'constitutes empiricism'. Along the way, the essays 're-use' (rather than 'apply') concepts from 'philosophy, psychology, semiotics, communications, literary theory, political economy, anthropology, Cultural Studies, and so on' (2002: 18).

Massumi calls his writing 'affirmative and inventive' (*pace* Colebrook and Deleuze quotes above), and links it to the humanities rather than the sciences, although this does not help the reader to find clear definitions in his work. He does, however, list a 'crowd' of words (that he calls 'concepts') that figure in some or all of his essays. The most ostensibly psychological, as we have seen, include: 'affect', 'perception', 'sensation', 'intensity', 'tendency', 'habit', 'movement', 'image', 'effect', 'force'. Indeed, he says (Massumi 2002: 19) that he wants to initiate a 'conceptual contagion', rather than try to 'get it right' (whatever 'it' may be), the later academic aim being an example of 'imperialist disciplinary aggression'. 'The project of this book is to explore the implications for Cultural Studies of th[e] simple conceptual displacement: body-(movement/sensation)-change' (2002:1). One way of understanding this abstract claim is to acknowledge that attending to 'sensation' and 'movement' within and of the body will re-orient bio-psychological theorizing towards 'change' (change, in general, as it were, not in relation to material objects and processes as they are spoken of, or assumed, in natural language.) Massumi opines that the humanities have ignored 'movement' (perhaps this is also inspired by Bergson):

> Attention to the literality of movement was deflected (in the humanities) by fear of falling into 'naïve realism', a reductive empiricism that would dissolve the specificity of the cultural domain in the plain seemingly unproblematic 'presence' of dumb matter. (Massumi 2002: 1)

So 'culture' (and for psychologists that would presumably include all social/human 'environment' or context) was seen as a 'mediation' occupying the 'gap between matter and systematic change'. Massumi jettisons this static, causal, and descriptively-prosaic account of sensations and other psychological processes and events in favour of post-structuralist metaphysics. Physicists and psychologists study 'dumb matter' or, he might imply, they study matter dumbly. Indeed, *Parables for the Virtual*, in Massumi's words, attempts to 'snatch experience from the jaws of science' (2002: 230).

It is important to note the metaphor for 'science' employed here: conventional science swallows reality as it tries to understand it. But Massumi wants to have his science and eat it too, by equivocating and obscuring the claims he makes about matter – matter that can be magically brought to life through his creative prose, it seems. Or perhaps he merely wants to retrieve experience philosophically, or, as is usually said in the humanities nowadays, 'theoretically'. He invites us to see 'philosophy' as a kind of 'wonder', so he presents a discussion of various questions around the body's responses to, and relationships with, what seem like unseen (or unseeable) aspects of sensory, perceptual and cognitive phenomena.

Ironically, Massumi sees his work as *anti*-metaphysical, even though he coins a register of terms that seem to refer to no objective reality. Indeed, he asserts that '[r]eality is not fundamentally objective. Before and after it becomes an object, it is an inexhaustible reserve of surprise' (2002: 214). What could this possibly mean? It slips between subjective and referential claims, and seems to postulate some event ('surprise') as the material forerunner of reality. He also claims that the abstraction 'relationality' exists 'over and above' actual relations (a Platonic universe, indeed!).

These are very metaphysical ways to avoid metaphysics. Other inconsistencies emerge through his essays, including the claim that he is not a social constructivist because he regards this position as 'deterministic'. Yet his own anti-determinism is very selective, and he allows, for instance, that 'in fact, certain normative progressions such as that from child to adult are coded in' (2002: 3). Without considering any more of Massumi's epistemologically evasive examples, it can be concluded that this highly-acclaimed writer presents what can only be judged to be counterproductive analyses on behalf of Cultural Studies' critique of academic psychology and of 'science' generally.

Realism as an Ethical Attitude

For those readers who have taken the pains to follow my analysis, let me review briefly the interests of this chapter. Theory-inspired Cultural Studies has proliferated often ill-defined concepts from phenomenology (following Bergson) via the self-proclaimed 'radical realism' of Massumi, who relies on Deleuze for much of his terminology. I have argued that this commits Massumi and his followers to a vitalist and non-deterministic 'neo- (or should that be 'pseudo-'?) psychology'. I see many of the analyses offered under the banner of Cultural Studies as purely verbal, lacking empirical implications.

Lest it be claimed that Theory is unconcerned with the questions on which academic psychology has focused since the end of the nineteenth century, I have quoted Blackman and Massumi in detail to demonstrate that the ambition of Cultural Studies has been to rewrite much of this field. To the extent that Theory presents metaphysics (and I have allowed relevant writers to proclaim this ambition in their own words), it attempts to undermine and then to transcend the tenets of scientific biological and social science. Blackman claims to deal with transdisciplinary studies that cross 'the borders and boundaries between psychology, sociology, cultural theory, anthropology and sociology [sic]' (Blackman 2008: 7). As we have seen, she rewrites several medical and psychiatric phenomena in order to show how humanities can illuminate the shadows of scientific ignorance (recall glycaemia as 'performance'). Similarly, Massumi's publicity refers to 'a new set of theoretical issues'; Cultural Studies offers 'potential new paths for the wedding of scientific and cultural theory'.

The kind of writing about psychological phenomena exemplified in this chapter probably discourages sceptical, empirical humility in the face of social and cultural complexity. It may have these effects simply as a result of its dense, vaguely-defined catalogue of novel 'concepts' (words?) used in eccentric ways. It is likely to deflate students' ambition because they cannot possibly emulate its ecstatic enthusiasm for 'levels of reality' and infra-empirical (does that mean unseeable or non-existent?) forces. Worse, perhaps, students might nevertheless gain the approval of their mentors by recirculating such arcane vocabularies, regardless of their reference to material reality, by invoking 'virtualities' and 'forces' or 'affect' as recommended by the exemplary Theorists.

Alternatively, students might judge that writing in this way amounts to little more than intellectual 'bluffing' because no public tests can be adduced by which to evaluate its truth (a provocative conclusion on which I will expand in the next chapter).

> Modern Psychology arose in part out of a justified criticism of contrived speculations that were never measured against any systematically constituted empirical domain ... All this does not mean that we should now replace naïve naturalism of the past with a simpleminded sociological reductionism. (Danzinger 1990: 194–5)

Massumi explicitly tries to replace contemporary Psychology's methodologies with his own. But I have found in the enthusiastic adoption of Francophone metaphysics only a misguided attempt to discard psychology along with 'naïve naturalism'. The Anglophone discipline, which had its roots in nineteenth-century natural science and in Enlightenment epistemologies, is increasingly seen by those trained in the humanities as trivially empiricist and individualistic (a point also made by Danziger). But the flight into post-structuralist phenomenological speculation has turned out to be embarrassingly ill-conceived. The annexation of psychological terms or *concepts* like 'affect' by post-structuralist Theory seems to be as arbitrary as it is idealist: reifications like 'intensity' as an 'emotional *state*', filled with 'vibratory motion', etc., do not clearly refer to any kinds of material processes or to specific mental phenomena, however much an author claims the status of a 'super-empiricist'.

As I have mentioned in previous chapters, Theory writing such as Massumi's is unapologetically psychological. It aims to reconfigure the 'nature-culture continuum' [*sic*], and 'will have a major effect on cultural theory for years to come'. Of course, the nature-culture question is the motivation for studying what has come to be known as academic Psychology itself. However, the affected metaphysics I have tried to understand in this chapter seems unlikely to incite students' curiosity about either nature or culture, let alone the details of how they interrelate. Worse, it discourages the very sense of wonder that Cultural Studies writers claim to want to provoke through their work; their openness to 'Theory' denies the value of theories. Yet the very epistemological realism that Cultural Studies derides presupposes humility in the face of contingency – an openness to discovering how things actually are independently of one's own expectations or interests:

> No world, no imagination. To imagine you need an external social situation and physical stuffs. In particular, art always comes from, uses, and returns to the real world. Realist art celebrates its own origin and return to the world and hence celebrates the world itself and our place within it. (Sartwell 2004: 12)

Similarly, for science. If my analysis has been fair, then post-disciplinary students are currently wasting a lot of precious time trying to emulate writers such as Massumi. They might be advised to read instead psychology or anthropology textbooks, even novels, which occasionally challenge their readers' attitudes to the value of knowledge. In Ian McEwan's *Saturday* an exasperated Dr Henry Perowne muses rather defensively that

> [a] man who attempts to ease the miseries of failing minds by repairing brains is bound to respect the material world, its limits, and what it can sustain – consciousness, no less. It isn't an article of faith with him, he knows for a quotidian fact, the mind is what the brain, mere matter, performs. If that's worthy of awe, it also deserves curiosity; the actual, not the magical should be the challenge … the supernatural was the recourse of an insufficient imagination, a dereliction of duty, a childish evasion of the difficulties and wonders of the real, of the demanding re-enactment of the plausible. (McEwan 2005: 67–8)

McEwan's grumpy scientist reminds us that 'realism' can imply an ethical perspective, not just an epistemological position.

Chapter 8

Theory and Education

You don't have to know this, you only have to learn it.
                                        Anonymous Australian University Lecturer, 2007

Man is the only animal that blushes. Or needs to.
                                        Mark Twain

Realism as a 'Default Position'

> One of the most striking features of recent discussions of the moment of theory is the lack of even proximal agreement about what the object of such theory might be and about the language in which it has been or should be conducted. (Hunter 2006: 112)

Ian Hunter notes that each of the older disciplines undermined (my word, not his) by the 'return of a certain kind of metaphysics to the Anglo-American academy' varied across 'disciplinary and indeed national contexts'. True though this may be, the specific *implications* of Theory demand analysis in relation to particular fields of enquiry – the established disciplines it casts aside. Hence the focus of this book has been limited to Psychology and its methodological contexts. Although seldom acknowledged as relevant to the 'Theory moment', a peculiar neo-psychology clearly permeates Theory-inspired curricula. Cultural Studies has emerged as a field that itself sometimes employs ad hoc empirical procedures, and, as we have seen in earlier chapters, purports to explain and interpret all manner of psychological as well as social and semiotic phenomena – from people's use of pornography to their emotional responses to family photographs and what it means to identify with an ethnically specific culture. So it describes 'real' people who enact (or are enacted through) 'culture', at least in part. It therefore makes claims that compete with theories and observations made within the established methodologies of psychoanalysis, cognitive and social psychology, and sociology. As we have seen, it even aspires to biological, including neuro-physiological, speculation.

Failing to learn from the Sokal Hoax and its aftermath, Cultural Studies' continuing recourse to European metaphysics has probably deepened the chasm between biological approaches to psychology on one hand and more socially-contextualized study of mind and behaviour on the other. Psychology, taught historically and methodologically (and therefore theoretically), survives in few humanities faculties in the new century. In the inter-, cross-, and post-disciplinary faculty, new methodologies have largely displaced twentieth-century academic Psychology. Culture abhors a vacuum: Cultural Studies curricula today incorporate much of what was once humanistic psychology and, of course, cultural anthropology. As Cultural Studies melds literary studies and theoretical sociology, especially, so it undervalues empirical, comparative sciences. What I have characterized as pseudo- or neo-psychology in this volume may be the only literature dealing with Psychology's traditional questions that humanities students will encounter in today's fragmented Arts curricula.

Cultural Studies has expanded to fill the gap left by Psychology's increasingly narrow definition of its field and methods as 'science' modelled on biology. Psychology has found a new home (and greater research funds) by relocating to the house of 'real', capital-S Science. In Australia and the United Kingdom a second change has occurred. Academic Psychology increasingly serves as education only for would-be professional psychologists: hence, it is in high demand by undergraduates and is becoming increasingly functional, clinical and 'applied'. Yet 'post-structuralist' Cultural Studies versions of Psychology do little to help students understand their actual selves or societies. Ironically its generalized abstraction and idealism obscure the conditions and the causes of human struggle, the conflicts, anxieties and pleasures of people's various cultural identities.

My critics might object that the Theory incorporated into Anglo-American Cultural Studies was never intended to provide alternative explanations of the phenomena that concern the traditional academic disciplines. It offers *critique* by rejecting the epistemological and ontological certitudes of the social sciences. As we have seen, however, many of its proponents writing in English *do* re-analyse and offer causal/explanatory accounts of psychological and social phenomena. Some of their accounts are proposed as alternatives to those of academic Psychology.

Hunter (2006: 83) points out that, with regard to Theory's 'posture of critique adopted in relation to so-called empiricist and positivist sciences', its strategy cannot explain why anyone would want, or need, to adopt its methods. To put his point in my terms, this is because writing such as Massumi's *mélange* of psychological terms and microbiology, for instance, only makes sense if the reader *already assumes* certain objective scientific knowledge (about the nervous system, genetics, etc.). Capital-T Theorists then embellish this assumed knowledge, but also proclaim it passé in the process. Theory does not present new empirical findings, new biological theorizations that clarify or systematize existing knowledge. And, of course, its proponents engage in no biological research as such. On the contrary, it simply (or tortuously) appropriates existing knowledge as a *pre-text* for writing creatively across disciplinary boundaries. So the claim to undermine the empirical knowledge of Psychology and to transcend it through the invention of hyperrealist (and vitalist) concepts is duplicitous at best.

Despite its claims to intellectual originality and profundity, Theory often means glossing terms from other scientific fields for no more than literary effect. Recall an example cited earlier in this book:

> There are few things all chaos theorists agree upon. One of them is that chaotic self-ordering depends on 'sensitivity to initial conditions', no matter how far the system has drifted from its initial terminus. What is this continued openness to being affected by a previousness of process? Is not this enduring 'sensitivity' a connecting thread of affect meandering impersonally through the world? World affect: life-glue of matter. (Massumi 2002: 227)

The author does not intend this way of putting words together to be read as mere poetry. It *refers* to something; it is *about* how the material world 'works', if we take the propositional import of the passage seriously. But what, exactly, can be meant by this shopping list of abstractions? How could students of Cultural Studies incorporate this mode of analysis into their methodological kitbag? How could they discuss this passage with any flatmates specializing in Geography or Geophysics? Could they believe or disbelieve what the passage seems to assert? Could any evidence be adduced to help them to decide whether 'affect' is the 'life-glue' of 'matter'?

When Theory writing challenges the way that established disciplines have analysed or described phenomena from their respective domains, there is often more than a hint of 'ontological envy' in its claims. The writers seem to want to 'own' the field, or, as Theorists themselves might say, to 'colonize it discursively'. We have seen many psychological-sounding proposals throughout this book that proclaim new knowledge but really offer little more than new words for older concepts. Of course, only a realist would make this criticism, for only a realist would think that the phenomena that writers seek to interpret and/or explain (yes, explain!) do actually exist *independently* of those who write about them, however lucid or obtuse their literary style.

I have argued that Theory writers in Cultural Studies offer few or no means by which students can evaluate their proposals. No methodological criteria are available to the novice other than those already practised within the fields that Theory rewrites, and Theory's proponents avoid making these explicit. So students are frequently intimidated into allowing methodological licence to Theory-speak because they lack the foundational knowledge that the established disciplines (especially analytical philosophy) might have fostered. They have to judge as empirical the kinds of Theory-drenched texts I have discussed throughout this book. They have no option but to take at face value Massumi's claim to be 'radically empiricist' and 'hyperrealist'.

Most students probably believe that people are not *tabula rasa*, and that human beings come into the world as a collection of certain species-specific qualities that are *causally relevant* to who and what individual people become. People are not infinitely plastic; they cannot tweak themselves into new futures voluntarily. It is not naïve or pre-theoretical for a student to believe that biology is a factor determining personalities, subjective identities. Not surprisingly, it has proven beyond the power even of Cultural Studies to educate students out of such beliefs. So a kind of ventriloquial hypocrisy is prominent in the contemporary academy: students are rewarded for mixing their epistemological claims willy-nilly, and they shift between folk-psychological beliefs and 'scientific' cause-effect assumptions and literary excess. If students are uncertain about how a sentence is meant to be read – is it metaphorical or is it literal – how can they evaluate the claim it makes?

In the interests of allowing students to contest the ideas of those writing or teaching Cultural Studies, I modestly propose that *all* participants in the relevant debates (all 'voices in the discourse') *explicitly define their terminologies*, including abstract and relational terms. I see this as a minimal condition for critical analysis. It would expose whether particular terms were meant to designate phenomena (or classes of phenomena) and whether particular propositions were being used to predicate qualities of them. It would allow the theoretical status of terms to be clearly agreed *before* hyperbolic claims were made using the concepts. Relations (such as 'difference') and processes (such as 'becomings') would not then be used to perform magical Theoretical tricks by being invoked at will, free of all specific material reference.

Fiona Hibberd shows that logical positivism, including its most luminous proponents, argued that some concepts could only be defined *implicitly* and did not 'point to real things'. She quotes Schlick who defends the non-empirical qualities of such implicit definitions:

> A system of truths created with the aid of implicit definitions does not at any point rest on the ground of reality. On the contrary it floats freely, so to speak, and like the solar system bears within itself the guarantee of its own stability. None of the concepts that occur in the theory designate anything real. (Hibberd 2001: 304)

Theorists and the post-structuralists whom they imitate seem unlikely to align themselves with the logical positivists, and indeed they claim that their epistemology is itself, in their particular sense of the term, 'realist' or even 'hyperrealist'. However, as Maze states:

> Realism founds itself … on the requirements of coherent, intelligible discourse. One of these, with wide ramifications, is the rejection of the concept of intrinsic or constitutive relations, that is, the notion that an entity can have its relations intrinsic to its own nature without any external correlative terminus. A relation can only be meaningfully spoken of as holding between two independent terms … We must speak of awareness as the awareness of something, but if the objects of our awareness exist only in our awareness of them, then there is no independently existing object of that relation. (Maze 2001: 395)

The requirements of coherent discourse are violated by the various writers I have considered in previous chapters in just the way that Maze identifies. They habitually postulate relations as 'intrinsic'. Indeed, they see this as a virtue, and call such relations 'immanent' without *referring to any entities* that could stand in *particular kinds* of relationships with each other. By contrast, unreconstructed realists recognize that *relations hold (or 'obtain') between and amongst entities and situations*. This does not commit realists to belief in platonic universals or in linguistic or mental idealism. As Hibberd (2001) asserts, realists accept that psychosocial events can only be understood in concrete, contextualized terms.

In short, realists value observation-based theorization of 'psycho-social events' of the kind of interest to Cultural Studies. Necessarily, realism is deterministic, but it need not assume some transcendental viewpoint, an omniscience 'above' actual situations – realism needs no god's eye view of situations. No 'transcendental' epistemology needs to be assumed to speak coherently about the psychological things also discussed by Cultural Studies.

Additionally, 'humanism' (Chapter 5), interpreted in a minimal and realist sense, can also be assumed without guilt. I do not mean by this that people should be seen as the centre of the universe or as having special status within a religious cosmology. Rather, Cultural Studies needs only to work with what is known about *people as a species*, as socially diverse, sociologically-embedded biological phenomena (like any other species). It goes without comment that, as a *culture-making* species, humans constitute a particular class of entities and possess certain qualities. Questions about their culture and nature are interdependent and can only be answered by empirical investigation. Theory may be of limited use in this regard.

I propose that realism be reinstated as the 'default position' in the humanities and social sciences at least until arguments to the contrary are built into the relevant curricula. In crowded and haphazard Arts and Social Science curricula, where Philosophy and Psychology may not form a central part of a student's experience, this seems reasonable. Where Cultural Studies or other interdisciplinary teachers introduce metaphysical critique into their teaching, it is only professionally responsible that the assumptions generally accepted in the established academic fields be presented clearly and subtly. This would allow competing analyses to be understood as just that – alternatives claiming to displace each other; alternatives amenable to argument. Generally, this would mean teaching students what various realisms claim and do not claim. At the very least it would ask for universal assent to the proposition that 'statements can refer unambiguously to states of affairs' (Hibberd 2001: 343). Otherwise, how is education possible?

A balanced, critical education would entail reading particular theories (in the plural) centred on 'the subject'. Realist empirical semiotic literature would need to be canvassed. Sophisticated alternatives that deal directly with the issues Theory tries to rewrite can easily be found. For example:

- Theo van Leeuwen's *Introducing Social Semiotics* (2007) presents a 'Functionalist' semiological model that detours around the metaphysical quicksand of European structuralism and post-structuralism.
- Petocz (1999) has written elegantly about Freud's theory of symbolism from a realist standpoint.
- Ian Hacking (1999) and Fiona Hibberd (2001, 2005) write on 'social constructionism', positivism and realism (within Psychology especially).
- Gavin Kitching's *The Trouble with Theory* (2008) uses Wittgenstein's analyses of linguistic 'knots' to straighten out Political Science students' idealist invocation of 'discourse' as an all-purpose material force. He gives sane pedagogical advice for dealing with the educational consequences of the mantra that 'discourse is power'.
- Roy Bhaskar has written extensively on 'critical' realism, provoking attempts such as Chouliaraki (2002) to synthesize his 'realism' with 'a constructionist' ontology.
- More successfully, a detailed, historically-situated critique of 'social constructionism' in Psychology (especially of Kenneth Gergen) is presented in Hibberd (2005, 2008). She

prescribes 'situational' realism (a version of direct realism) as an antidote to relativist epistemology.
- Bell and Staines (2001) canvass the conceptual and methodological hurdles that confront Psychology students, including issues centred on definition explanation and measurement, again from a realist position.
- Alan Wolfe's *Human Difference: Animals, Computers and the Necessity of Social Science* (2003) discusses humanism and its critics within the discipline of Sociology, while at the same time cautioning against positivism and scientism.
- Michael Lynch's *True to Life: Why Truth Matters* (2004) lucidly discusses truth, relativism, and epistemology. He considers the epistemological and educational importance of retaining a non-relativist notion of 'truth'.
- *How the brain creates the self* is addressed by the neurologist and psychiatrist Todd E. Feinberg in *Altered Egos* (2001). His account is 'relational' or 'ecological' (in the sense discussed in this book) and explores the paradoxes of Cartesian dualism, so it is anything but philosophically naïve. Feinberg's highly readable book is broadly realist in its approach.

These writers are not familiar to Cultural Studies teachers. Perhaps this is because each considers seriously what I have called the realist 'default position' in relation to the epistemological and psychological assumptions debated in the humanities and social sciences. For example, Lynch points out that the notion that propositions can be judged objectively true or false (at least in principle) is tacitly assumed even in the writings of those whom English-language Theorists claim as their epistemological mentors, such as Michel Foucault:

> The real problem with ... relativism is not that it misdescribes our concept of truth. The real problem is that it pulls the rug out from under the feet of any attempt to rationally criticise the political system of power in one's own culture. (Lynch 2004: 39)

For the realist, 'rational criticism' is central to a liberal-arts education. Those engaged in debate need to accept the requirement of logical consistency, and so agree that determinism, cause-effect relationships, objectivity, etc. are necessary starting points for contesting each other's claims. Good faith is also essential. This involves giving to one's interlocutors clear definitions of one's own terminology and assumptions, and, of course, sincerely *believing* these oneself. Believing a statement usually means judging it to be true, so the arbitrary postulation of hidden forces and powers (such as 'God's will' or 'virtual' relations) to 'win' arguments would be illegitimate in rational discourse of the kinds that I believe teachers are professionally bound to encourage.

My criteria for genuine debate may sound like common academic sense. However, many university teachers in today's post-disciplinary fields of study are openly sceptical about some or all of my demands. Some are scornful of appeals to 'reason' or 'logic' ('they're just social conventions', it is asserted, even of Aristotelian logic). Others are antagonistic to science in general, which they see as politically repressive (hence the culturalist analyses of biological research on gender, genetics, etc.). Because Cultural Studies also analyses the social contexts of scientific and hermeneutic practice, it deals critically with the politico-cultural significance of the humanities themselves. Its curricula and textbooks include a wide range of epistemologies united only in being anti-realist and sceptical about the established sciences. Theory writers central to Cultural Studies frequently purport to unmask ideological and metaphysical subtexts of the physical as well as the social sciences. So the possibility of sedate debate about the matters canvassed in this book seems as remote as it is necessary if post-disciplinary education is to challenge students rather than train them to reject without argument whole fields of knowledge and the epistemologies that underpin them. 'Textualism' quickly becomes a vicious circle, whether in the (post-)humanities, or in recontextualizing the propositions contested within what were once called Sociology and Biology.

When Students 'do Theory'

It is ironic that Enlightenment liberalism motivated Cultural Studies' turn away from the empirical disciplines of the post-war university. So, despite my criticism of Cultural Studies' metaphysical novelties, I want to stress that I have little problem with the proliferating analyses of actual cultural practices, with semiotics in general, or even with attempts to clarify what concepts like 'subjectivity' and 'difference' mean in particular contexts. But, surely, sub-fields of Cultural Studies such as 'Queer Theory' have no need to imply a *metaphysical* revolution. The growth of political critique and identity studies centred on race or gender 'difference' is irrelevant to my attempt to restore coherence to these debates. I remain sanguine about the mundane and quotidian neo-anthropology that makes up much of the Cultural Studies field.

My concerns are *methodological* and *therefore* educational. As a tertiary teacher I assume that students of Arts and Social Sciences come into the university expecting the humanities to explore what used to be summarized as 'the human condition' (or better, 'conditions'). They should be curious, excited by the prospect of *discovering* facts and *conceptualizing* how to interpret what human cultures and societies do, and how they create meaning for their members – people's various histories, identities, experiences and political conflicts. That Cultural Studies claims to 'radically decentre the human subject' must come as an educational shock to many a hapless student. Like me, they might ask whether English versions of European metaphysics are necessary or helpful for an education that revolves around *cultural* questions. So I ask:

- Do students of Cultural Studies need to accept the kinds of metatheoretical and conceptual novelties I have canvassed in this book? How could these help them to understand human psychology, different societies, or the why and how of cultural forms and practices?

- Does assuming that 'becomings', and not 'things' or situations, are the furniture of the universe really matter to a student analysing the ethical engagements invited by *Big Brother*?
- Does the unreconstructed Kantian subject silently lurk in the subtext of all those essays penned by undergraduates who remain unenlightened by Theory?
- Is Cartesian dualism eradicated by recourse to the insights of 'Body Theory' (Blackman 2008)?
- Does 'affect' actually permeate the material world as well as the psychological realm? If so, must a student develop the skills necessary to detect its power and to write elegantly about it? How is 'affect' related to bio-psychological concepts, to 'pleasure' or 'pain'?
- What are the implications of postulating as psychological 'entities' such free-floating reifications as 'intensities', 'excesses' and 'potentialities'?
- Where do literary and poetic discourses meet the objective and the scientific? Or, more appropriately, why should the former be seen as alternative, indeed better, ways of writing about material cause-effect relationships?
- Should not all students be taught to examine critically, rather than to accept on trust, Theory's claims to displace the objective and empirical discourses of the humanities and social sciences?

These are *educational* issues. They are difficult to address without sounding censorious, or worse. However, I want to argue that, insofar as it claims the academic high ground in regard to realism and to humanism generally, 'Theory' should, at least, be taught *dialogically*: curricula must allow students seriously to explore the traditions and methodologies of the social and psychological sciences that are said to be transcended by Theory's metaphysics. Not to do so is to short-change our students.

The rhetorical Theory that I have confronted throughout this book has made even the Foucault-inspired 'discourse fever' of the 1980s and 1990s seem clear-headed and sociologically engaged by comparison. As a humanities teacher I have been continually disappointed by the intimidated confusion of students who borrow metaphysical jargon and try to write in the style of Deleuze or Massumi. Unfortunately, it is only the most able postgraduate student who manages to weld into some kind of linguistic cohesion the disparate, poorly-defined terms that Cultural Studies uses to 'rethink' Theory. The jargon may be sourced from Neuroscience, Biology, Zoology, or Psychology. Sometimes it seems that the main purpose of essay and thesis writing is simply to 'do Theory' – to coin new definitions and invent novel contexts for established concepts, to celebrate words invented to redescribe empirical phenomena, without leaving the security of the computer. Here is an instance from a thesis about the (admittedly very complex) relationships between people and technology. Taking up the question of 'the body as subject', and borrowing from Massumi the concept of 'potential', the postgraduate writes:

> Rather than placing one body as primary to the assemblage we can think of the body as an intensely connected node in a distributed network of sometimes realised, but never

wholly contained, potential. The subject is defined by this dynamic network of intensely realised and externally contingent potential.

The supporting analysis for this interim conclusion in the student's argument is equally abstract and, like the above, it outlines in general terms how the human species uses tools that become extensions of the body, and vice versa. This student wants to take the human out of the grammatical subject position in his analysis, presumably because that would posit the body as a causal agent in the process being theorized (recall Chapter 6). Like his mentors, he emphasizes an abstraction, 'relationality':

> ... the non-specificity of culture or species in technical development (the emergence of technical archetypes across cultures) combined with the evidence of a correlative cortical development only indicates their codetermination. It doesn't indicate that either cortical or technical development determines the development of the other. The incipiencies realised between the 'naked' human and material world are indeed determined via a 'direct emanation of species behaviour' (Steigler, 1998, p. 154). But as a 'direct emanation' the tool thus becomes a part of the body – or rather the material of the tool and the body become the basis for a technical assemblage, a codetermination. The value of Leroi-Ghouran's zoological approach to technics lies in the realisation of this codetermination between body and world'.
>
> For Steigler this means that a second type of memory augments and modulates genetic memory. However, the memory of the stereotypes lies not only in the mind/body of the human but also in the material trace of the technical artefact itself.

A number of things strike the reader about this kind of writing. The most obvious is its register of technical terms, some more or less defined, others not. To be fair, the writer footnotes 'incipiency' as 'an already beginning to happen', from the *Oxford English Dictionary*. But he seems ill at ease with many of the other words he employs. He has to revert to more or less common usage in order to convey his Theoretical take on tool use. So, alongside 'assemblages' and 'distributed networks of potential', other registers are invoked ('species', 'cortical development', 'memory stereotypes') although each is given its own particular connotations in the passage. Still, the writer must rely on the common understanding of these non-Theory terms for the paragraph's apparent coherence.

Second, the ambition of the student to take on matters of metaphysical moment is impressive. Some might even find it startling, given that many postgraduate theses are timid and narrow. But whether judged brave or foolish, this passage is undeniably intellectually serious and the writer is attempting to work at a high level of abstraction. To the uninitiated, reader, however, the most notable aspect of the passage is this: unless the reader already accepts its mode of analysis as methodologically valid, they can learn nothing from it about anything in particular. One can admire its elaborate redefinition and recontextualization of everyday terms. One can marvel at the metaphysical system this presupposes (indicated by terms like 'assemblage' and 'subject'), by which to analyse how people and tools/technologies form ensembles. One might well agree that such processes cannot be understood other than interactively or ecologically, if I may paraphrase. Yet the passage sounds hollow because it refers only to abstractions. 'Codetermination', 'genetic memory' and 'technical archetypes' would presumably be defined elsewhere in the student's work, but, like the references to 'cortical development' and 'the material trace of the artefact', they seem little more than scientific-sounding rhetoric. In this respect, the writing resonates sympathetically with examples I have considered throughout this book. It invokes phylogenetic biology, bodies, tools etc., and it seems empirical enough. It proposes causes and effects; its proponent might even label it 'hyperrealist'.

My second (again anonymous) example of unnecessary metaphysics is by another postgraduate, who writes, inter alia, that 'every action is perpetually in the service of two functional and co-present phases: the abstract phase of immanent potential and the actual or concrete outcome of these immanent relations'. These phases and outcomes are bodily; that is, they occur in actual things that people recognize as their bodies – 'the real-material-but-incorporeal ... the body as a positioned thing', she writes, citing Massumi's paradoxical phrase. Without asking the obvious questions about the ontological status of this set of constructs, it may be sufficient to note here that the student's topic is the institutional and aesthetic 'place' of Internet art in the contemporary exhibition environment. Why she needs to stumble over eccentric metaphysical postulates in order to get a grip on the 'real-material-but-incorporeal' is anything but obvious.

Teaching Theory

Teachers of Media and Cultural Studies who expect conceptual subtlety backed by rigorous empirical analysis from their students are increasingly dismayed by what passes for research in their field. For them, the passages discussed above will sound tendentious. They appear unnecessarily abstract, pretentiously so. The style seems designed to elevate the writers above the very materiality they purport to reconceptualize. Theory seems to be a way of avoiding the topic at hand rather than engaging with it, even if it does provide a sense of omnipotence in the face of recalcitrant reality.

The literary theorist Terry Eagleton saw the obsession with the 'signifier' and 'discourse' that found its flag bearers in Derrida and Foucault during the past two decades as a retreat from political engagement by humanities scholars. In an age of consumer capitalism and the failure of the utopian left, he comments:

> The freedom of text or language would come to compensate for the unfreedom of the system as a whole. There would still be a utopian vision ... [One could imagine] that utopia had already arrived in the shape of the pleasurable intensities, multiple selfhoods and exhilarating exchanges of the marketplace and the shopping mall. (Eagleton 1997: 22)

Confronted with the fact that the humanities (and the post-humanities) are fast becoming educationally irrelevant, Cultural Studies offers no resources for resistance. The 'Theory Wars' (or whatever the media now call them) have compounded the devaluation of humanities education across the board. Despite the rise and rise of Cultural Studies, Arts degrees have seldom enjoyed less prestige or had less relevance to the political and cultural life of the communities in which they are earned.

Clearly, the fragmentation and atrophy of the humanities and social sciences result from many factors – economic, political and educational. However, the concurrent retreat into metaphysics seems unlikely to provide a positive example to the detractors of literary, historical or cultural scholarship. In faculties where industrial-strength abstraction and obscurantism have found so ready a market, how can one foster the intellectual modesty necessary to explore and discover things about what it means to be a person? If, from the very early stages of their education, students are confronted with dismissive and grandiose claims about the traditional humanities, how will they develop confidence to enter into the debates du jour? Educational engagement is unlikely if students are asked to assume that Theory's new armoury has already destroyed the Anglo-American psycho-philosophical canon, the adherents of which are now seen as trudging interminably through the mire of anachronistic realism, burdened by the dead weight of the Enlightenment.

Bluffing

The educational consequences of Theory-speak have been largely negative for Anglophone education. Generally speaking, yoking metaphysics to post-disciplinary studies has meant that what were once philosophical questions have been moved sideways into new fields where they are little understood. The principal result is that the revised Theory merely intimidates most students. Having to pretend to understand that the 'subject' is a semiotic chimera is likely to produce a sense of cynical disempowerment in a sociology student interested in social class, gendered power, or why Fascism has not died long after the Third Reich. Celebrating cultural diversity as 'difference' offers no insights into cultural conflicts and their complex histories; theorizing 'identity' is largely irrelevant to understanding or criticizing religious fundamentalism or the politics of Internet pornography. Students simply do not understand why novel ontological speculation, 'process metaphysics', 'affect' or 'intensities' and other reifications (which are often presented as ways of overcoming reification, indeed) should be essential to their various liberal arts educations.

As one who has tried to guide students methodologically, I would make a stronger claim: *Many students who have been rewarded with high grades for employing the terminology of Theory cannot even be said to understand it. They are not able to draw from the literature they cite specific implications that have empirical or conceptual import.* I have taught many able students who cannot make coherent propositional sense of the very Theory that they quote in their essays and theses.

Students are frequently rewarded for writing in purely literary ways, for invoking concepts of Theory only for their vague, rhetorical connotations. In earlier chapters I considered the Deleuzian notion of 'becoming' as a noun. This term confounds students wishing to incorporate it into English language sentences. This is because what I call the default position in modern education (above) involves accepting *that real objects and processes can be referred to* using language, and 'becomings' seems to form a new ontological class entirely. Unless they imbibe the whole of French post-structuralist philosophy, students will have to take refuge behind quotation marks placed around terms such as these. They will hope to be rewarded for invoking 'becomings' in their essays, though they may never have heard of, let alone endorse, process metaphysics.

'Affect' is a similar educational hurdle that needs to be overcome. As we saw in earlier chapters, this term is often used to label a peculiarly *factotum,* vitalist concept. It points to something ineffable about reality, something that science and folk psychology alike have overlooked. This is especially problematic if a student has been trained to accept that words sometimes or usually *designate situations or phenomena in the world,* but finds that 'affect' seems not to refer to any psychological quality or phenomenon at all. In this case all the undergraduate can do is write as though 'affect' is just a free-floating stylistic option, referring to nothing actual. Its use simply shows they have read the literature imposed by their teacher. If they do this, the student is surely bluffing. The teacher has not demanded intellectually-rigorous work, only a display of the linguistic badge necessary to claim membership of the 'Theory-club'.

Post-Humanities and Education

The edifice of twentieth century Anglophone humanities appears to be crumbling from within. Although the university may not yet be 'in ruins' (Readings 1996), the disciplines on which Anglo-American Arts faculties were centred have become fragmented and unfocused: their teaching terms have been reduced, assessments are frequently trivialized (exams have virtually disappeared), and research methodologies are increasingly marginalized within undergraduate curricula. These morale-deflating trends have been obscured by the growth in humanities research and publication, often in new online journals designed for those writing in post-disciplinary ways about culture, politics, sociology, semiotics, or niches within these fields.

Like their science colleagues, humanities and social science academics are forced to compete viciously for research funding. Teaching quality is supposedly evaluated by bureaucratic means, by questionnaires and quantification. However, in the absence of any demonstrable improvement in pedagogy, let alone in the quality of, say, senior undergraduate theses (a benchmark of Australian tertiary education) students have become almost as cynical as their teachers. Many now attend university as infrequently as they can, while simultaneously grasping employment opportunities in the 'real world' – the world that sees little value in education unless it leads to a professional qualification. So Law and vocational degrees in media studies, journalism or communication are increasingly favoured by the most successful school-leavers.

In the corporatized and competitive university, academics increasingly work from home, reducing the likelihood of inadvertent intellectual conversation on campus. When was the last time a lecturer bumped into a student on the library steps and ended up spending an hour talking about Cambodian politics or the 'digital divide'? None of this is due to moral failure in either the lecturer or the student, of course. It is the result of the complex processes that are transforming the Anglophone university. The disciplines that are grounded most deeply in the English language and its cultural contexts have faced the most profound challenges from these rapid changes in the student body and in students' study practices. I will not discuss these here, other than to suggest that the apparent educational democratization effected in the name of Cultural Studies needs to be seen in the context of the fragmentation and casualization of Anglophone humanities education during the past two or three decades.

The Cultural Studies child was born out of well-founded criticisms of its humanities parents: if History was too narrowly Eurocentric, study other cultural formations; if Psychology had become scientistic and objectivist, revert to other paradigms like phenomenology; if Sociology had been trivialized and seemed like an apology for functionalism and political conservatism, then look to European semiotics and 'structuralism' for a new discourse. Yet the emerging pluralist field betrayed its Anglophone roots by seeking to justify *in the most general and abstractly metaphysical terms* its so-called *anti*-foundational, founding assumptions. As evidenced throughout this book, by the 1990s, Anglophone Cultural Studies was increasingly written in the lexicon of French 'post-structuralism'. A normalizing vocabulary emerged within which to conduct conversations about the object of study – culture. Moreover, culture had come to mean more or less anything previously studied under the names of humanities or social science anyway. Therefore students seeking an education in Cultural Studies found they had to understand the older humanities anyway, if only to transcend them by performing Theory-based critique.

Theory had become an end in itself. 'More Theory' was the call from Cultural Studies teachers, although what the hapless student might have thought this meant is anybody's guess. Students were asked to show metaphysical originality even if they could not spell 'epistemology' and knew nothing about the arguments for and against observation-based methodologies in the social sciences. They sometimes wrote in explicitly anti-realist ways, even while tacitly accepting realist epistemology in every other part of their lives and education. Many completed their degree without *testing* the revolutionary epistemologies and process ontology implied by Theory. Ignoring Aristotle, Hume, Weber, Parsons, Freud, Levi Strauss, even de Saussure, most read only glosses, deconstructions and travesties of foundational humanities and social sciences literature.

As pretentious as it is tendentious, Theory's implied neo-psychology impedes contemporary humanities education. It angers the most able students and bores many others made subject to its opaque discourses. Its becomings do not become it. Whatever its newly-minted ontologies, they can only make sense to undergraduates and professors alike if the disciplines they discard and the philosophical concepts they purport to displace are also understood in their respective historical contexts.

Recall that a leading Cultural Studies academic defined the field as

> a way of contextualisisng texts of any kind – of analysing the social relations of textuality; and there's no reason why it shouldn't include literary texts and literary regimes amongst its proper objects of knowledge ... It shifts the interpretive gaze from a self-contained text to its discursive and social framings, within which students are themselves implicated; while at the same time it opens up potentially fruitful methodological exchange between distinct protocols of interpretation that apply in the social sciences and textual disciplines. (Frow 2006)

However, as we have seen, Cultural Studies often breaks out of these intersecting circles of textuality. It *does* make claims about the *nature* of the social and psychological world, about human thought or perception, about evolutionary adaptations, about epistemology, chaos theory, even about genetics and particle physics. At least implicitly, it boasts that these are *competing proposals* about *what is the case in the world*. How else could an undergraduate understand, say, a cultural rather than a biological claim about peoples' 'racial' or 'gendered' identities? In short, Theory-inspired post-disciplinary writing makes claims that seem *empirically contestable*, and not merely *hermeneutically contestable*. However, interpretation and 'analysis' can only be contested if their terms *refer to real phenomena or to other theories that do so*. Educationally, this needs to be acknowledged so that evidence can be debated (although evidence would not be the only matter at issue, of course).

As I have shown, and as even Colebrook and Massumi occasionally admit, Theorists' discourses are not merely *textual* in the sense of, say, biblical exegeses or literary criticism. The Theorists I have discussed certainly do not think they are writing astrology or theology. Yet undergraduates can be forgiven for confusion on this point: Theory-laden Cultural Studies is all too often presented as though no procedurally-explicit, publicly-repeatable methods are appropriate to critically evaluating its statements, even when they sound like factual propositions to the undergraduate in search of an example for their essay in *Cultural Studies 101*. By contrast, realists would challenge students to ask whether Theory's own assumptions should be accepted as *true*, its various arguments as valid or invalid. Undergraduates would need not only to defend their beliefs, but also to justify their choice of conceptual vocabulary.

I am not confident that many Theorists would accept and debate my methodological and pedagogical proposals. They might complain that I had missed the point: those who adopt Theory do so for 'political' reasons, they would say. 'Theory' is a postmodern way of being 'left-critical'; epistemology has nothing to do with this. For instance, Greg Hainge writes that Lou Reed's 'anti-music' can be thought of as an exemplary model for Theory, which he equates with '*the philosophical practice proper to that discipline*', i.e. to Cultural Studies of a Deleuzian kind. If one accepts this recommendation literally, then a non-ideational cultural form (music) is being proposed as a method for verbal analysis to imitate. Predictably, he dismisses Sokal and Bricmont's *Intellectual Impostures* as 'fairly puerile', and rather cryptically warns that it

> will continue to pose a threat to the future of Cultural Studies and Theory as disciplines [*sic*] within an increasingly rational, corporate academic climate that responds to market forces and suffers the use of science-based models within the humanities only when it comes to funding criteria. (Hainge 2002: 296)

He proposes a second methodological metaphor for the 'proper' (i.e. non-rational, non-scientific) approach to studying culture, one that he hopes will avoid the 'static, enclosed forms such as that of the circle' and lead instead to 'dynamic forms that enter into becomings'. However, like the students struggling to write Theory whom I have quoted in this chapter, he himself resorts to ontologically-banal 'objects' and 'things' anyway: 'Cultural Studies and theory must be anchored in the real since they can only exist as a challenge to the real' (2002: 297). Left-critical philosophy, therefore, involves 'challenging the real'. On this account its politics centre on ontological questions. I will resist the temptation to parody this paper and merely point out that it appeared in a refereed international journal, *Continuum: Journal of Media and Cultural Studies* (on the editorial board of which I once served).

As also discussed in Chapters 1 and 2, what Cultural Studies theorists propose by 'challenging the real' is nothing short of a newly-minted 'ontology of the social':

> It is difficult to overstate the scope of Deleuze and Guattari's challenge to social theory. What they propose is nothing less than a new *ontology* of the social, of social being, grounded in a philosophical ontology of *Being as pure difference or becoming*. Being, for Deleuze and Guattari, is that which differs from itself, *in nature*, always already, in itself, qualitatively different. (Bogard 1998: 53, emphasis in original)

Again, relational terms are reified wantonly to produce sentences that sound grammatically well-formed but are likely to flummox the average undergraduate (and their grammar-check). A few pages later, Bogard (1998: 57) writes that whereas most sociological theory highlights exchanges – of money, women, gifts, etc. – 'society is not about exchange but about the articulation and disarticulation of libidinal energies'. So the old-fashioned 'real' gets smuggled back in as 'desire', although 'desires are not formal, interchangeable units, but dynamic connections of bodies that vary in intensity and composition'. (Fortunately, Sociology students are seldom asked to understand colonialism or world poverty in terms of the curiously disembodied becomings and other articulations of libidinal energies.)

No Laughing Matter

I have argued that a highly abstract strand of neologism, vitalism and reification continues to intimidate humanities undergraduates a decade after Alan Sokal so publicly embarrassed the intellectual impostures of Theory. Many humanities academics still lament the Enlightenment, which they believe continues to imprison twenty-first century students in structures of reason, committing them to essences and objects, rather than celebrating the liberating potential of processes, articulations and change. The humanities and social sciences stand accused of ignoring the vital forces that animate our becomings. By contrast, post-disciplinary metaphysics promises to free undergraduates from the straitjacket of rationality and realism.

A decade ago, reading Sokal and Bricmont's exhibits of metaphorical befuddlement was fun, but the joke is now wearing thin. Most Cultural Studies academics have resolutely avoided the implications of the exposé. So the fabric of Anglophone humanities is still creased by anti-realist conventionalism (Kitching 2008) and by vitalist metaphors that students can do little more than unknowingly parody. Meanwhile, those of us who believe that some propositions refer to actual entities and situations have modestly to decline neologistic invitations to 'perform' alternative ways of 'doing and thinking knowledge'. Instead we can only plead that, as Cultural Studies has pitched its marquee on the ruins of the disciplines through which it has wielded its elegantly designed wrecking ball, realist methodologies should continue be taught explicitly, critically, and in good faith.

Like all fields of academic study, Psychology is enriched by deep knowledge of its history and methods (including the competing methodological issues raised by its diverse theorizing). Similarly, Cultural Studies' Theory and its epistemological dilemmas can be taught dialogically, by argument and counter-argument. Theory could then legitimately claim its place in today's crowded curricula. To do this, Theory teachers will at least need to ask: *why should students believe some arguments and not others?* Can some analyses *justifiably* be preferred to others? These questions might be expected to unite Theorists and their more empirically-minded colleagues in a common educational enterprise. To the realist teacher something important remains at stake in modern academic analysis and argument, something more than optional ways of speaking: to educate our students we have to accept that some statements can *reasonably* be claimed to be *true or false*. So we should be prepared to state clearly why we think some propositions must be judged to be meaningless. Educationally, however, this is a difficult challenge. As John Searle recently commented, 'It is much easier to refute a bad argument than to refute a truly dreadful argument' (2009: 89). And, despite the warnings of the Sokal hoax, Cultural Studies' Theorists continue to celebrate some truly dreadful arguments.

References

Barker, C. (1999) *Television, Globalisation, and Cultural Identities*. Milton Keynes: Open University Press.
Barthes, R. (1973) *Mythologies*. St Albans: Paladin.
Bell, P. & Staines, P. with Michell, J. (2001) *Logical Psych: Reasoning, Explanation and Writing in Psychology*. Sydney: UNSW Press.
Bell, P. (2003) 'Neo-Psychology Or Neo-Humans? A Critique of Massumi's Parables for the Virtual', *Continuum: Journal of Media and Cultural Studies*, 12: 4, pp. 445–82.
Berkeley, G. ([1710] 1998) *A Treatise Concerning the Principles of Human Knowledge*. J. Dancy (ed.). Oxford: Oxford University Press.
Berlin, I. (2004) 'A Letter on Human Nature', *New York Review of Books*, 23 September, 26.
Bernardi, D. (2002) 'Cyborgs in Cyberspace: White Pride, Pedophilic Pornography', in J. Friedman (ed.) *Reality Squared: Televisual Discourse in the Real*. Piscataway, NJ: Rutgers University Press.
Bhaskar, R.A. ([1975] 1997) *A Realist Theory of Science*. London: Verso.
Blackman, L. (2008) *The Body – The Key Concepts*. Oxford: Berg.
Bogard, W. (1998) 'Sense and Segmentarity: Some Markers of Deluzian-Guattarian Sociology', *Sociological Theory*, 16: 1, pp. 52–4.
Bullock, A. & Trombley, S. (eds.) (2000) *The New Fontana Dictionary of Modern Thought*. London: HarperCollins Publishers.
Butler, J. (1990) *Gender Trouble: Feminism and the Subversion of Identity*. London: Routledge.
Chouliaraki, L. (2002) 'The Contingency of Universality': Some Thoughts on Discourse and Realism', *Social Semiotics*, 12: 1, pp. 83–111.
Colebrook, C. (1999) 'A Grammar of Becoming: Strategy, Subjectivity, and Style', in E. Grosz (ed.) *Becomings: Explorations in Time, Memory and Futures*. Ithaca: Cornell University Press, pp. 117–45.
Colebrook, C. (2002) *Gilles Deleuze*. London & New York: Routledge.
Cultural Studies Association of Australasia (2003) Culture Incorporated: Bodies, Technologies, Habitats. *Culture 2003 Conference Abstracts*. Christchurch: Cultural Studies Association of Australia/Christchurch Arts Centre.
Crandall, J. with Niva, J. (2005) ;Between Movement and Position: Tracking and Its Landscapes of Readiness', *ephemera: theory and politics in organisation*, 5: X, December http://www.ephemeraweb.org/journal/5-X/5-Xindex.htm. Accessed 7 August 2008.
Danzinger, K. (1990) *Constructing the Subject: Historical Origins of Psychological Research*. Cambridge, MA: Cambridge University Press.
Deleuze, G. (1978) *Lecture Transcripts on Spinoza's Concept of Affect*, 24 January, http://www.webdeleuze.com/php/sommaire.html. Accessed 3 November 2008.

Deleuze, G. (1986) *Cinema One: The Movement*, translated, H. Tomlinson & B. Habberjam, Minneapolis: University of Minnesota Press.

Deleuze, G. (1990) *The Logic of Sense*, translated, M. Lester with Stivale, C., C.V. Boundas (ed.), New York: Columbia University Press.

Deleuze, G. & Guattari, F. (1987) *A Thousand Plateaus: Capitalism And Schizophrenia*. Translated and Foreword by Brian Massumi. Minneapolis: University of Minnesota Press.

Dennett, D. (2005) *Sweet Dreams: Philosophical Obstacles to a Science of Consciousness*. Cambridge, MA: MIT Press.

Despret, V. (2004) *Our Emotional Make-up: Ethnopsychology and Selfhood*. NY: Other Press.

Durand, J. (1970) 'Rhetorique et image publicitaire', *Communications*, 15, pp. 70–95.

Dyer, R. (1997) *White: Essays on Race and Culture*. London: Routledge.

Eagleton, T. (1997) *The Illusions of Postmodernism*. Oxford: Blackwell Publishers Ltd.

Eco, U. (2000) *Kant and the Platypus: Essays on Language and Cognition*, translated, A. McEwen. New York: Harcourt Brace.

Erasmus, D. ([1509] 2008) *Praise of Folly*, translated, R. Clarke. Richmond, UK: Oneworld Classics.

Feinberg, T.E. (2001) *Altered Egos: How the Brain Creates the Self*. Oxford: Oxford University Press.

Franklin, J. (2000) The Sokal Hoax and Postmodernist Embarrassment, *Continuum: Journal of Media and Cultural Studies*, 14: 3, pp. 359–62.

Freud, S. (1976) *Jokes and Their Relation to the Unconscious*. Harmondsworth: Penguin.

Frow, J. (2006) 'Literature, Culture, Mirrors: John Frow Responds to Simon During', *Australian Humanities Review*, http://www.australianhumanitiesreview.org/emuse/culture/frow.html. Accessed 3 November 2008.

Genosko, G. (2003) 'Introducing Deleuze' Review Essay of Claire Colebrook (2002) *Understanding Deleuze*, Sydney: Allen & Unwin, *Cultural Studies Review*, 9: 1, May, pp. 224–28.

Grant, R. (1996) 'Anti-Meaning as Ideology: The Case of Deconstruction', in A. O'Hear (ed.) *Verstehen and Humane Understanding*. Royal Institute of Philosophy Supplement, 41: Cambridge University Press, pp. 253–85.

Griffiths, P. (1997) *What Emotions Really Are: The Problem of Psychological Categories*. Chicago: University of Chicago Press.

Grosz, E. (ed.) (1999) *Becomings: Explorations in Time, Memory and Futures*. Ithaca: Cornell University Press.

Guattari, F. (1995) 'On Machines', tranlated, V. Constantinopolos, *Journal of Philosophy and the Visual Arts: Complexity: Architecture/Art/Philosophy*, 6, pp. 8–12.

Hacking, I. (1999) *The Social Construction of What?* Cambridge, MA: Harvard University Press.

Hainge, G. (2002) 'A Whisper or a Scream? Experimental Music Sounds a Warning for the Future of Theory', *Continuum: Journal of Media and Cultural Studies*, 16: 3, pp. 285–98.

Harraway, D. (1991) 'A Cyborg Manifesto: Science, Technology and Socialist Feminism in the Late 20th Century', in D. Harraway *Simians, Cyborgs, and Women: The Reinvention of Nature*. London: Free Association.

Hawkins, G. (2006) *The Ethics of Waste: How We Relate to Rubbish*. Sydney: UNSW Press.

Hayles, N.K. (1999a) *How We Became Posthuman: Virtual Bodies in Cybernetics, Literature, and Informatics*. Chicago: University of Chicago Press.

Hayles, N.K. (1999b) 'Simulating Narratives: What Virtual Creatures Can Teach Us', *Critical Inquiry*, 26: 1, pp. 1–26.

Hibberd, F.J. (2001) 'Gergen's Social Constructionism, Logical Positivism and the Continuity of Error. Part 2: Meaning as Use', *Theory and Psychology*, 11: 3, pp. 323–46.

Hibberd, F.J. (2005) *Unfolding Social Constructionism*. New York: Springer.

References

Hibberd, F.J. (2008) 'Situational Realism, Critical Realism and the Charge of Positivism'. Paper submitted to *History of the Human Sciences*, May 2008.

Hirsch, E. (1982) *The Concept of Identity*. New York: Oxford University Press.

Hodge, B. (1999) 'The Sokal "Hoax": Some Implications for Science and Post-Modernism', *Continuum: Journal of Media and Cultural Studies*, 13: 2, pp. 255–70.

Hunt, D. (1997) *Screening the Los Angeles "Riots": Race, Seeing and Resistance*. New York: Cambridge University Press.

Hunter, I. (2006) 'The History of Theory', *Critical Inquiry*, 33, Autumn, pp. 78–112.

Kitching, G.N. (2008) *The Trouble with Theory: The Educational Costs of Postmodernism*. Crows Nest, NSW: Allen & Unwin.

Kurtzweil, R. (1999) 'I Process Binary Opposites, Therefore I Am', *Black + White*, 36, April, pp. 25–6.

Lynch, M.P. (2004) *True to Life: Why Truth Matters*. Cambridge, MA: Cambridge University Press.

MacCormack, P. (2001) Becoming Human: Deleuze and Guattari – Gender and Third Rock from the Sun, *Intensities: The Journal of Cult Media*, 2005, 1, Autumn.

MacCormack, P. (2002) 'Barbara Steele's Ephemeral Skin: Feminism, Fetishism and Film', *Senses of Cinema*, September, http://archive.sensesofcinema.com/contents/02/22/steele.html. Accessed 3 November 2008.

McEwan, I. (2005) *Saturday*. London: Jonathan Cape.

Massumi, B. (2002) *Parables for the Virtual: Movement, Affect, Sensation*. Durham, NC: Duke University Press.

May, T. (1997) *Reconsidering Difference: Nancy, Derrida, Levinas, and Deleuze*. University Park, PA: Pennsylvania State University Press.

Maze, J. (2001) 'Social Constructionism, Deconstruction and Some Requirements of Discourse', *Theory and Psychology*, 11, pp. 393–417.

Milner, A. & Browitt, J. (2002) *Contemporary Cultural Theory*, 3rd ed. Crows Nest, NSW: Allen & Unwin.

Monk, R. & Raphael, F. (eds) (2001) *The Great Philosophers*. London: Phoenix.

More, M. (1994) *On Becoming Posthuman*, http://www.maxmore.com/becoming.htm. Accessed 3 November 2008.

Murphie, A. (1997) 'Putting the Virtual Back into the VR', *Canadian Review of Comparative Literature*, XXIV: 3, pp. 713–42.

Murphie, A. (2005) *Differential Life, Perception and the Nervous Elements: Whitehead, Bergson and Virno on the Technics of Living*, http://www.culturemachine.net/index.php/cm/article/viewArticle/32/39. Accessed 18 September 2009.

Murphie, A. & Potts, J. (2003) *Culture and Technology*. New York: Palgrave.

Neville, A.O. (1947) *Australia's Coloured Minority: Its Place in the Community*. Sydney: Currawong Publishing Co.

Nietzsche, F. ([1883–1885] 2006) *Thus Spoke Zarathustra: A Book for All and None*, A. Del Caro & R.B. Pippin (eds.) Cambridge: Cambridge University Press.

Petocz, A. (1999) *Freud, Psychoanalysis, and Symbolism*. Cambridge: Cambridge University Press.

Pinker, S. (2008) 'Goodness, Gracious Me: There is Scientific Evidence that Evolution has Endowed us with Ethical Impulses', *The Sydney Morning Herald*, 2–3 February, Spectrum, pp. 26–7.

Rassos, E. (2006) Questions of Temporal Presence and Absence in Contemporary Film and Video. UNSW: PhD Thesis.

Readings, B. (1996) *The University in Ruins*. Cambridge, MA: Harvard University Press.

Redding, P. (1999) *The Logic of Affect*. Ithica: Cornell University Press.

Rich, F. (2008) 'How to Cover an Election', *New York Review of Books*, 29 May, 55: 9, pp. 9–10

Rose, S. (2005) *Lifelines: Beyond the Gene*. London: Vintage.
Rostand, J. (1967) *Inquiétudes d'un Biologiste*. Paris: Gallimard.
Russell, B. (1961) *History of Western Philosophy*. London: George Allen & Unwin.
Rutsky, R. L. (1999) *High Techné: Art and Technology from the Machine Aesthetic to the Posthuman*. Minneapolis & London: University of Minnesota Press.
Ruthrof, H. (2000) *The Body in Language*. London: Cassell.
Sartwell, C. (2004) *Six Names of Beauty*. New York: Routledge.
Schatzki, T.R. (2002) *The Site of the Social: A Philosophical Account of the Constitution of Social Life and Change*. University Park, PA: Pennsylvania State University Press.
Schirato, T. & Yell, S. (2000) *Communication and Cultural Literacy: An Introduction*. 2nd ed. Crows Nest, NSW: Allen & Unwin.
Searle, J.R. (2009) 'Why Should You believe It?' *New York Review of Books*, 24 September, 56: 14, pp. 88–92.
Shouse, E. (2005) 'Feeling, Emotion, Affect', *M/C Journal*, 8: p. 6, http://journal.media-culture.org.au/0512/03-shouse.php. Accessed 3 November 2008
Sokal, A. & Bricmont, J. (1998) *Intellectual Impostures: Postmodern Philosophers' Abuse of Science*. London: Profile Books.
Thrift, N. (2004) 'Intensities of Feeling: Towards a Spatial Politics of Affect', *Human Geography*, 86: 1, pp. 57–78.
Van Leeuwen, T.J. (2005) *Introducing Social Semiotics*, London: Routledge.
Wetherell, M. & Potter, J. (1992) *Mapping the Language of Racism: Discourse and the Legitimation of Exploitation*. London: Harvester Wheatsheaf.
Williams, R. (1981) *Culture*. Glasgow: Fontana Paperbacks.
Wolfe, A. (2003) *Human Difference: Animals, Computers and the Necessity of Social Science*. Berkeley, CA: University of California Press.

Index

aesthetics 89, 90
affect 89–104
   'affection-image' 91–92
   'affectus' 90, 93, 97

Barker, C. 51, 53, 64–65
Barthes, R. 21, 22, 58, 89
Becoming 32–33, 49–51, 60–61, 98; *See, also* Blackman, Colebrook, Deleuze, Despret
begging the question, examples of 9, 50, 53, 60, 64, 65, 69, 78, 103, 111
Bell, P. 55, 56, 69, 116, 130
Berkeley, G. 87
Berlin, I. 7
Bernardi, D. 77
Bhaskar, R.A. 129
Blackman, L. 100–103, 107–113, 120–132
Bogard, W. 19–20, 32, 139
Body Theory 32, 101, 103, 111–113, 132
Bricmont, J. 25–27, 34, 36, 37, 39, 139, 140
Browitt, J. 25–26
Bullock, A. 75, 113
Butler, J. 7, 60, 64–66, 68

causality 35, 94
   biological causality 107
   quasi-causality 94
Chouliaraki, L. 129
chaos theory 35, 39, 138
'Clever Hans' 101–104
coherence, as logical requirement of discourse 9, 83, 131–133
Colebrook, C. 23–24, 33, 38, 46–51, 60, 78, 80, 84, 93, 118, 138
Cultural Studies Association of Australasia 60

Crandall, J. 95–96, 98
culture, defined 20–21
   culturalism 62, 67–68, 69
cybernetics 38, 78, 84
cyborg 76, 77, 79, 81–82

Danzinger, K. 121
Deleuze, G. 15, 19, 23–25, 31–39, 47–51, 56, 58, 80, 84, 90–93, 95, 96, 98–99, 113–116, 118, 120, 132, 139
Dennett, D. 95, 116
Despret, V. 101, 109
disciplines, academic 17–19, 22, 24–25, 37, 39, 43, 49, 59–60, 69, 107–108, 125–127, 131, 136–139, 140
   post-disciplinarity 8, 9, 21, 33, 35, 37, 45, 108, 121, 125, 130–131, 135, 136, 138
Durand, J. 58
dualism 103, 109, 110
   Cartesian Dualism 69, 101, 108, 130
Dyer, R. 51

Eagleton, T. 33, 62, 67–68, 108, 134
Eco, U. 59
education 125–140
emergence 58, 63, 78, 80, 84, 94, 133
emotion 36, 60, 68, 95, 102, 109, 121
   and 'affect' 15, 89–93, 96–97
empiricism 48, 52, 55, 58, 99, 115–119
   hyper-empiricism 117
Enlightenment 74–76, 121, 131, 135, 140
   post-Enlightenment 19, 21, 61, 73, 83, 114
episteme, definition of 83
Erasmus, D. 15
essentialism 45–51, 54, 76, 107, 110–111
   and race 51–54

ethics 44–45, 74–76, 83, 98, 112, 120–122
evolution 45–46, 69, 76–77, 80–81, 114, 138
'excess' 95
explanation 25, 43–47, 55–56, 68–69, 101–103, 110–111, 130
and interpretation 24–26, 43, 45, 55, 59
extropians 81

Feinberg, T. 69, 130
foundationalism (epistemological), avoidance of 98–99; *see also* 'becoming(s); ontology
Franklin, J. 33, 34
free will 62
Freud, S. 7–8, 68, 74, 89–90, 98–99
Frow, J. 24–25, 138

gender/sex 64–65, 85, 110
  essentialism and gender 58–59, 64–67, 69; *see also* essentialism
  feminism 26, 58–59, 65
  gender 22, 27, 46, 76, 77, 78, 82, 131
  gender identity 22, 59, 61, 62, 64–67, 138
  gender as 'subject position' 63
  masculinism 25–26
Genosko, G. 23–24
Grant, R. 48
Griffiths, P. 68
Grosz, E. 99–100
Guattari, F. 19, 21, 32, 34, 63, 93, 98, 115, 139

Hacking, I. 129
Hainge, G. 31–32, 138–139
Harraway, D. 76, 77, 81
Hawkins, G. 98
Hayles, N.K. 60, 75, 76, 78, 81–82, 84
Hibberd, F. 10, 49, 83, 128–129
Hirsch, E. 68
Hodge, B. 33, 34
homo sapiens 79, 80
humanism(s) 22, 60, 73–76, 78, 81, 83, 108, 114, 129, 132
humanities 16–20, 26–27, 125–140
  new humanities 35, 107
  post-humanities 135, 136–139
  see also post-humanism

Hunt, D. 52
Hunter, I. 125, 126
hypoglycaemia 111

identity 51–56, 59–70; *see also* gender/sex

Kitching, G.N. 129, 140
Kurtzweil, R. 77

Lynch, M.P. 130

MacCormack, P. 78
McEwan, I. 122
Massumi, B. 16–17, 22, 31–35, 37, 46, 48–49, 78–81, 84, 90, 94–98, 107, 113–121, 126–127, 132, 134, 138
May, T. 47
Maze, J. 94, 128
metaphor, theory as 33, 35–36, 38–39, 78, 85, 94, 98, 119, 139, 140
Milner, A. 25–26
Monk, R. 90
More, M. 80–81
Murphie, A. 36–38, 55, 77, 81–82

neuropolitics 95
neurology 69
neurophysiology 95, 107
Nietzsche, F. 71, 80–81

ontology 47–56, 89–100

performance, body as 100–104, 107, 111–113, 120
Petocz, A. 129
phenomenology 27, 43, 80, 91, 95, 97, 107, 108, 113–118, 120, 121, 137
  defined 113–114
Pinker, S. 45–46
positivism 48, 58, 128, 129, 130
post-humanism 73–85
postmodernism 9, 34, 138
Potter, J. 52–53, 56
Potts, J. 46, 57, 77, 81–82
process ontology 51, 91, 99, 108, 137

Index

race/racism 51–56
Raphael, F. 90
Rassos, E. 93
Readings, B. 136
Redding, P. 89
reductionism 8, 27, 44, 45–47, 67–69, 110, 111, 121
realism 48, 49, 50, 53, 94, 99, 119, 120–122, 125, 128–132, 140
    as 'default position' in education 9, 129, 130, 136
    hyper-realism 27, 97, 107, 126, 127, 128, 134
reification (of concepts) 23, 45, 48, 56, 82, 83–84, 90, 92, 95, 97, 107, 121, 132, 135
    defined 94
Rich, F. 100
Rose, S. 46–47
Rostand, J. 29
Russell, B. 13, 114, 116
Rutsky, R.L. 82
Ruthrof, H. 63

Sartwell, C. 105, 121
Saussure 58, 59, 137
Schatzki, T.R. 75–76
Schirato, T. 64, 65–66
schizophrenia 21, 23, 67, 93, 110
    as 'dementia praecox' 110
science 107–122
'Science Wars' 26, 33
Searle, J.R. 77, 140
selective serotonin re-uptake inhibitors (SSRIs) 112

semiotics 59–67
    functional semiotics, see van Leeuwen
    literary semiotics 21, 58; *see also* Barthes, Saussure
Shouse, E. 96–97
Sokal, A. 25–27, 33–39, 97, 114, 125, 139, 140
Sokal Hoax 33–35, 39, 125, 140
Staines, P. 55, 56, 69, 130
structuralism 48, 129, 137
    post-structuralism 16, 32–33, 34–35, 37, 48, 58, 62, 80, 84, 114, 119, 121, 126, 128, 129
subjectivity 27, 60–70, 74, 79, 99, 60

textualism 131
    textuality 9, 24, 138
theory (capital-T) defined 16–20, 27
Thrift, N. 95–97
'the virtual' 35, 38, 50, 80, 94, 99–100, 115, 118–119
    virtuality 50, 78, 94, 95, 99
    virtual reality 114
Trombley. S. 75, 113

Van Leeuwen, T.J. 129
vitalism 90, 96, 113–116, 140

Wetherell, M. 52–53, 56
Williams, R. 21
Wolfe, A. 130

Yell, S. 64, 65–66